HERBAL

RITUALS

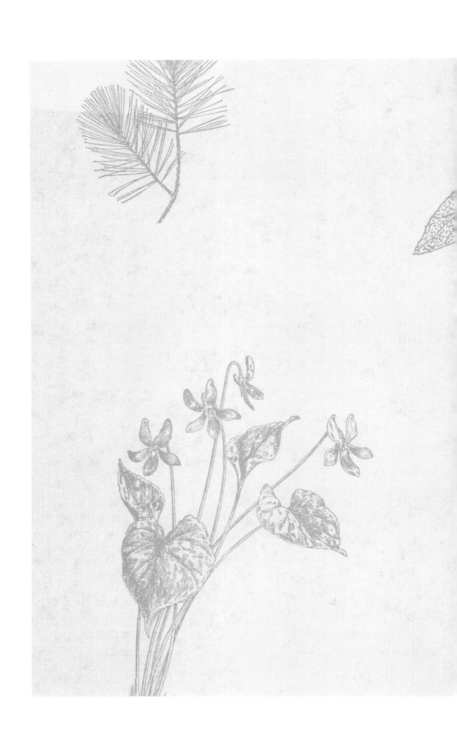

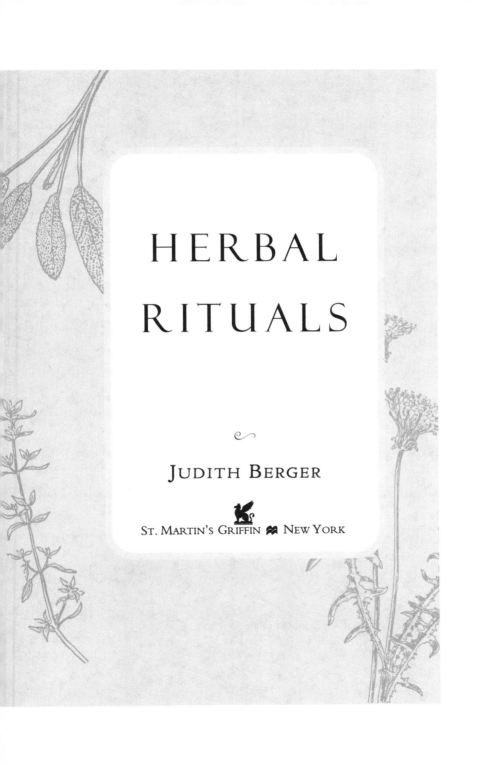

HERBAL RITUALS

Judith Berger

St. Martin's Griffin ✹ New York

To Tom and Hannah, for believing,
and to the earth, water, fire, and air for continuing

A Note to Readers

HERBAL RITUALS. Copyright © 1998 by Judith Berger. All rights reserved. Printed in the United States of America. No part of this book may be used or reproduced in any manner whatsoever without written permission except in the case of brief quotations embodied in critical articles or reviews. For information, address St. Martin's Press, 175 Fifth Avenue, New York, N.Y. 10010.

Library of Congress Cataloging-in-Publication Data

Berger, Judith (Judith L.)
  Herbal rituals / Judith Berger.
    p.   cm.
  Includes bibliographical references.
  ISBN 0-312-19281-9 (hc)
  ISBN 0-312-24301-4 (pbk)
  1. Herbs. 2. Herbs—Utilization. 3. Herbs—Folklore. 4. Herbs—Therapeutic use. 5. Cookery (Herbs) 6. Nature craft. I. Title.
SB351.H5B395 1998
581.6'3—dc21
                                                              98-34277
                                                              CIP

First St. Martin's Griffin Edition: September 1999

10 9 8 7 6 5 4 3 2 1

ACKNOWLEDGMENTS

LISTING THE NAMES of all those who have contributed in some way to this book just touches the gratitude I feel for the ground of support which was created by the presence of these people in my life. I am deeply grateful to all those who had a hand in keeping me well-nourished as I labored to birth this book, and to you all, I give heartfelt thanks:

To the divine messenger Denise Sylvestro, for planting the seed and to Kat Egan for insisting and making sure, that blustery January day at Benny's, that I watered the seed. To Tom Colchie, from the furthest reaches of my heart, for guiding me every step of the way and holding my hand when necessary, and to Elaine Colchie for her womanish encouragement and editorial assistance. To Michael Denneny for saying yes. To all of my herb teachers, especially Robin Rose Bennett, Kate Gilday, Susun Weed, Matt Wood, and Don Babineau, and to all my herb students for tromping out to the fields with me and being delighted about the weeds. To Clarissa Pinkola Estes and Father Matthew Fox for their inspiring, strengthening work. To Thich Nhat Hanh for his smile. To Elizabeth Hurst in Edinburgh for her faith and love. To Katherine Spiratos and Tad Wanveer for their healing hands. To Genevieve Kapuler, most excellent and inspiring yoga teacher. To the kids and staff at the A.C.T. program at the Cathedral of St. John the Divine for remembering the names of every plant I showed them and for eating them all. To the patient staff at the Cornell Medical Library, especially Patricia Tomasulo, Ani Khoubesserian, Kevin Pain, Jeanne Strausman, and McEvoy Campbell. To Michael Burns, for his computer assistance. To Citi Bakery for organic oatmeal, every day. To the founders and members of the Sixth Street and Avenue B garden for creating and maintaining that miracle. To Hannah Kirschner and Marisa DeDominicis, most deeply, for sewing, listening, feeding, mothering, sistering, and making much of the work-in-progress. To Jeanne Liotta for meals, late-night telephone venting, good sense, and every winter solstice. To Chloe

Liotta-Jones for hugs when most needed. To all my yoga students for being a welcome diversion from the computer screen. To Christine Kerrigan for helping me continue to teach as I wrote. To Noonie Marx and Eliot Stewart for demanding progress reports. To Brian Thomas for humor at the right moments. To Melody Doves, Naomi Eshler and Ilana Storace for reminding me of what I was doing. To Liza Lauber and Dale Bellisfield for reading sections of the work. To Harriet McCaig, Celia Brown, and Sarah Lewis for helping me keep the holidays. To Jane Wylie Potter Thornquist, bodhisattva of compassion and song sister, for Rilke and cookies. To Birgit Staudt for giving me courage. To Kathilyn and Piotr Probosz for hospitality. To Christina Huber and Darryl for helping me get off-island to the woods and water. To Mia and Madeline, Kali, Lucca and Selene, Akiva, Hillel and Yehudah, and Michelle. To Michael and Ellie Berger, for conversations about Halachic Judaism. To Mom, Dad, and Shari, for being proud.

Lastly, and with much devotion, I hug the trees for hugging me all these years and reminding me that there is always more than meets the eye. I kiss the earth in thanks for being so beautiful and inspiring, and the herbs for the magic and medicine they bring. To the blue spruce for sheltering me, the willow tree for whispering, and the elder, for hearing. May we all, always, be surrounded by the soul of nature.

CONTENTS

INTRODUCTION

WHEN I WAS a young girl I learned that the Brooklyn neighborhood in which I lived was called Midwood. My mind immediately and emphatically swept away all the neat row houses with their front lawns and driveways and conjured up a dark, evergreen forest in which giant trees bore themselves proudly, protecting the few hidden dwellings with their long, solid trunks. Ribbons of smoke plumed the treetops, rising from the chimneys of these old stone homes. When I discovered that Brooklyn had, just one hundred years earlier, been farmland, I saw myself standing beside my horse, upon a ridge, arms folded and feet planted, surveying a horizon bordered by pastures of grazing sheep.

Although I was raised in an urban environment, nature somehow burrowed its roots quite forcefully into the ground of my imagination. In truth, at the time they seemed exactly the same: Both nature and my imagination were unconfined, limitless in possibility. As a child I knew that if I looked at a leaf long enough, a miracle was sure to take place right before my very eyes. All the books I admired agreed with me; they confirmed the existence of trolls, dwarves, fairies, and witches with pictoral renderings and vivid tales. I spent a good bit of time hunting for these creatures beneath mushrooms and in the sidewalk cracks. So when a lone yellow blossom grew tall out of a fissure in the cement, I assumed it was the handiwork of elves and dropped to the ground, peering beneath the plant's basal leaves just in case I might spy a fairy wing. If I grew silent and cocked my ear toward the bee in the peony's pollen-drenched center, I might hear bee-speech in the sound of the drone. If I left the right gift—a penny, a song, a thimble full of water—a plant might even give me its name.

Needless to say, I skipped along the driveway and through the neighbor's yard in a constant state of anticipation that bordered on ecstasy. I never lost faith because it was not faith that drove me: It was certainty, and the excitement of the quest. My eyes became skilled at spotting the oak between buildings, the red berries in the yew hedge, at gazing into a net of branches to find the camouflaged nest, all as I waited for mom to pick me up from school.

Though one might have augured that I would make my home in a valley of lush greenery, what has always been familiar and comfortable to me is seeking out the green amid concrete surroundings. Encountering and attending to nature in the city fulfills my early childhood requirements for treasure: That it must be sought, recognized, and earned before it will reveal its name and the full measure of its richness.

It was destiny that led me to love the wild weeds enough to seek their names even as I planted myself in Manhattan, island of stubborn, urban beauty. Much of my apprenticeship in the craft and art of herbalism took place in Central Park's meadows and brambles, where my teacher taught me how to become silent and listen as the trees, shrubs, and herbs whispered their names into the wind. Alongside these excursions into the field were hands-on experiments in inventing and preparing different unguents, teas, powders, and mixtures from roots, leaves, berries, flowers, and seeds we gathered.

A curious feeling accompanied my studies: That I was remembering rather than learning this ancient knowledge. A sense of familiarity and peace enveloped me each time my fingers plucked berries and sorted seeds—valuable states in our chaotic, speed-addicted world.

Visiting the herbs in all weathers I began to notice not only their metamorphosis from week to week, but a distinct moodiness on the part of the environment which I came to sense through seasons of harvesting my own small store of medicine plants. I became aware of the presence of aliveness and sensuality in the air and earth that seemed to seek my attention and grow stronger upon having it. I found I could absorb this changing temperament by simply clearing my mind as I walked down a city street and focused on the intensity or dullness of that day's light, on the weight and smell of water in the air. The atmosphere seemed to possess a highly expressive nature which encircled my body like threads of smoke, summoning a torrent of images as I went about my business.

To settle my attention upon the elements in the city gave me the pleasurable experience of living in several worlds at the same time. Further, I found that the earth revealed, through its rhythms, an entire cycle of emotions and energies to which all creatures inhabiting her body responded. The human family seems unique in its neglect of this rhythm; it appears we have been away from home for too long, and have become technologically encumbered and mesmerized.

Practicing this contact makes the magic of nature available to us even as we go about our mundane lives. I believe an intimate connection with the earth and herbs, as beings of ever-unfolding mystery and delight, provides us with a sense of enchantment quite necessary to the life of the soul. Receiving this gift requires that we slow down, indeed, that we stop and breathe in the magic taking place around us all the time.

This book marks a single year's journey into the earth's cycles wherein we can explore our own generative and declining rhythms that move in conjunction with those of the land. Each monthly section offers the reader a doorway into the labyrinth of birth, growth, fruition, decay, death, and regeneration. The constant presence of the elemental world and the herbs can be used as a touchpoint to bring both body and soul back to an instinctive, strengthening rhythm.

While one may initially be drawn to a plant because of an ailment, one need not be ill to use any of the herbs highlighted in this book. Regular use of many of the herbs discussed will tone even a robust body. The recipes described in each chapter are offered to support playful physical contact with the herbs and foster the sensual component of herbal medicine. Gathering with others to brew concoctions of all kinds is a priceless balm for the isolation and poverty of spirit we sometimes experience in the modern age.

The rituals described in this book are offered as a means of directly touching the sacredness of nature. Watching the moon, soaking in an herbal bath, saving and using the seeds of vegetables we have eaten to mark new beginnings become, with our intent, magical activities. These simple acts draw us into the crests and dips of the yearly cycle while satisfying the child in us.

In each chapter, as you enter the waxing and waning patterns of nature's seasonal character, you may find yourself magnetically drawn outdoors, into the elements. Stand with your feet rooted to the earth, your face open to the wind, rain, sun, or moon. Listen closely, for you may hear a call, and if you heed this call you may be led closer to your instincts, dreams, and desires. For it is the voice of our beloved, breathing earth which is beseeching us, as it sways between rest and action, death and renewal, to join all creatures of the natural world in this spiral dance that refreshes us when we are parched and, even after the longest winter, always brings spring.

NOVEMBER

❧

Visioning, Dreaming, Remembering

AS A WILDCRAFTER, one who seeks out the plants on their home ground, respectfully gathering them for food and medicine, my very fingertips are in physical touch with November's gifts of coldness and death. This month brings with it a frequently lusterless sky and biting chill that keens through grove, forest, park, and street, a whistling canticle of winter's swift descent over the land. As I assemble my tools— knife, rootdigger, and spade—in the small willow basket which also contains a small pouch of cornmeal, I toss in my wool gloves with open fingers and cloak myself warmly to bear the sting of the wind which I know will dog my face during the hours outdoors.

Harvesting in November brings one into conscious contact with a retreating, somewhat unyielding earth, and with a heightened awareness of the growing slenderness of resources. The hardening ground requires that I increase my labor if I am to pull roots from her body, for she has contracted, clasping with passionate force tubers, corms, and rhizomes close to her breast, where an invisible, underground heart pumps warm life into the roots of plants and trees all winter long. As I part the rosebush branches I must sharpen my eyes in the grey pallor of winter's light and reach in deeply to find hips that have not yet taken on the shriveled countenance of the death-crone.

Aware that from Halloween onward, the plants are tended to by the winter gods and goddesses who inhabit the realm of shadow, I stand motionless before each plant or tree, closing my eyelids and asking silent permission to take herbs of utmost necessity; the late arrival of a first frost may have delayed the passage of vital force into the berries of bushes and roots of wild weeds, leaving me only this small window of time in which to gather particular, oft-used sources of medicine.

Returning home, I place my basket on the kitchen table and make myself some tea, thawing my hands around a mug of pungent thyme. Then I lay out the red-bordered linen towel which was my grandmother's, emptying the contents of my basket onto it and sifting carefully through what I have harvested, choosing for medicine those berries which are red and smooth-skinned, signs that they still carry the life and power which will enter the bloodstream of an individual and bring healing. I place clusters of plucked rosehip berries into jars and pour apple cider vinegar to cover them, my thoughts racing to the day I will twist the lid open and dip teaspoons into the tangy vitamin-C rich vinegar, using the brew to flavor soups while increasing my resistance to winter flus.

The concentrated, repeated movement of my hands from basket to cloth to jar relaxes and settles my body, quiets and entrances my mind, and soon my perception retreats to a place of vision in the back of my head. There I see a forest where the trees have become skeletons, standing tall in the dying November daylight, their opaque winter trunks now the yellow and ivory of bones, spines clacking a percussive, ancient rhythm as they sway with each blasting November gust. A moment later my vision returns to the checked tablecloth, with its cherry-edged, worn napkin and red berries, strewn into a pattern I feel certain some rag-wrapped, old-country women of my Russian-Lithuanian ancestry could read my future from. Swallowing a draught of tea, I continue my work.

VISIONING

The closed portal that seals the realm of ancestors and spirits from the material world remains unhinged between Halloween and the Winter Solstice, leaving us in a place where the past, present, and future whirl together. This time strongly magnifies our opportunities to connect with the voices of our ancestors, to call upon our dreams for guidance, and to open our intuitive ears for signs and portents which lead us toward new beginnings as we grope through this dark cycle of the seasonal year. The death-crone wraps, turns and tosses us in her shroud, rocking us toward inarticulate, dimly lit places in the mind beyond our conscious, everyday reach. It is within these cavernous, shadowy alcoves of the psyche that the crone has kindled fires, illuminating the treasures of self-trust, inner counsel, and renewal, the hidden gifts of this outwardly still season.

Amongst witches, November is the ripest month for gazing into the future or retrieving unwritten wisdom of ancient ways. The sensitivity and thinning of boundaries between the world of spirit and matter which many women experience psychically during their menstrual time is mirrored during this month; one's perception or sensation of either visually or aurally living simultaneously in several worlds increases. For myself, the month of November has become anchored to my relationship with my paternal grandmother, Lilian, who passed over at the age of ninety-two in 1989.

My five-foot tall grandmother had sturdy legs, a hearty laugh, and though she worked as the main breadwinner in her home while raising two children, she maintained an optimism and affectionate warmth toward all she came in contact with. For the last thirty years of her life, after her husband's death, she lived alone, contentedly, in a Brooklyn apartment, taking her daily walks in the below-freezing temperature she called "brisk weather."

My grandmother was an adept at solitude. Though she grew blind from cataracts in the last years of her life, she held her vision and sense of us firmly in the stout hands and keen nose which became her sources of vision. The Saturday she died, I was driving around Lancaster, Pennsylvania, and was suddenly struck with an urgent need to return to the city rather than stay in the country overnight. My partner and I, having had our fill of bleak November sky, made our way back to New York. When I arrived home, there was a message scrawled on paper for me: *Call home when you get in.* Even as I picked up the phone and dialed my parents, I knew she had died, peacefully, in her house. After weeping on the telephone with my father I sat down and drew a picture of her, dressed in the pink, thin-strapped, full-length slip she had given me on a recent visit.

Several weeks after her funeral, I accompanied my father to grandma's apartment to pick out some of her things for keeping. Drawn to her vanity, I opened a drawer, in which I found her rhinestone-beaded, cat's eye reading glasses; a black and white cameo necklace on a string of glinting jet beads; and an old, yellow cardboard shaker bottle of Jean Naté talcum powder. In her closet I found a pearl and green beaded evening bag; I put two pairs of ivory-colored crocheted gloves and a faded chiffon handkerchief into it. My grandmother's spirit felt alive in all these things; even the pair of mahogany bedroom night tables that flank my bed today make me feel protected in the circle of her love.

Each November, for the sake of remaining forged with my matrilineal lines, and for asking Lilian's assistance in visioning the future, I lay these articles out on the altar. The reading glasses, thanks to my cats, are now broken in two, and arch like blue-rimmed, tilted almonds on each end of the cloth-covered table. Some ebony beads, loosened from the cameo necklace, roll underneath furniture legs, to be found during a vigorous spring sweeping.

All cultures and spiritual traditions which employ the practice of visioning use objects or symbols as touchstones for spirit to enter, for the energies of matter and spirit to unite and create opening. Mirrors, stones, candle flames, tea leaves, and bowls of water are some of the substances and natural symbols which have been used for centuries to read the future. The natural mingling of the worlds of spirit and form in the dark time of the year also magnifies the possibility of successfully retrieving wisdom regarding the future from the spirits of our ancestors, whose sight extends beyond the human perceptive capacities nurtured in American culture. This time of the year, as nature is stripped to bareness, teaches us that simplicity, quiet, and rest create a gentle and powerful foundation for being able to set foot on the island of far-vision. A placid state of mind allows us, as Native American tradition aptly describes it, to "enter the void."

When I am seeking guidance, I sit before my altar and clutch grandma's black and white cameo in my hands, the jet black beads sparkling. For the past five years, on November 1, the Mexican Day of the Dead, my grandmother's spirit and I have become comfortable with a particular ritual. On that day, I pray and meditate, calling her to me with the cry only a grandchild knows how to make and a grandmother immediately recognizes. Responding to my call, grandma appears to me in some way and whispers a word or phrase into my ear; her words become a focus for me for the entire year. Following a time in which I had endured much suffering and loss, I heard her gently, and with much tenderness, say the words "you may begin again."

According to the Celtic calendar, November is the first lunar month and belongs to the birch tree, the tree of beginnings. I find it important that the beginning time is situated at a moment when nature has ceased any outward signs of growth and has plunged its vitality underground. From nature's rhythm I learn that beginnings extend their tethers from an invisible core or seed that germinates best in the ground of dormancy and otherworldly visions which accompanies this month. The dropping temperatures encourage our bodies to rest, to enter the realm of sleep, so that the unconscious can send us information for our growth through the messenger of our dreams. The herb I have chosen for this month is under the dominion of the Crone and has an extraordinary place in the world of plants as an enhancer of dream-life, in addition to the many physical strengths it offers our bodies.

MUGWORT *(Artemisia vulgaris)*

According to herbalist Maud Grieves, mugwort is said to have derived its name through its use in flavoring beer prior to the the introduction of hops. Mugwort's latin name, *Artemisia vulgaris*, invokes this plant's ties with the ancient moon goddess Artemis; in various clay figurines she appears with a hundred breasts, symbolizing the abundant well of nurturant power within her body which makes her capable of giving suck to the forest animals. Other representations of Artemis depict her as archer, a bow in her hand, the circlet of a crescent moon crowning her brow. These articles symbolize the moon goddess's sovereign role as protector of forest creatures, as well as holy huntress of those who threaten the sacred balance of her forest and as wise bringer of death.

The curved moon upon her brow, Artemis also appears as a numinous deity calling our attention to the holiness of the moon and the cyclical, lunar pullings which hold all earthly beings to an ever-returning spiral of life, death, and rebirth. Artemis offers women especially a potent image of female solitude which encourages us to wander, sure-footed and alone, as a way of centering and grounding ourselves, renewing our strength just as the blood-rich lining of our wombs replenishes itself with each full lunar transit. *Artemisia vulgaris* holds these qualities within her stalks, leaves, and roots, acting as a powerful ally for women seeking ancient, woman-defined attributes of female power.

Mugwort's renown among common folk as a powerful systemic healer reaching into the reproductive, digestive, urinary, and respiratory tracts has earned this artemisia the nickname cronewort. Like the old woman who has passed through many moons, harvesting wisdom into the folds of her wide skirt, this common weed, denounced and torn up recklessly by the ignorant, truly walks and lives amongst the people. As the village midwife once nurtured the heart of the community with compassion, knowledge, common sense, and magic, cronewort has soothed the pain of childbirth, eased the tenderness of aching joints, comforted bellies, and instilled vision among human beings for centuries with her knowing medicine.

Intractable and sturdy as a hag, cronewort stretches its roots amid those urban places humans tend to scurry rather than wander in, their hurried pace forgetful of the very existence of the natural world. Affectionately referred to in Russian as *zabytko*, which means forgetful, cronewort's strong camphorlike oils, when inhaled, open up chambers of ancient memory within the brain, bringing to one's dream life stirring visions of past and future that overflow with magical imagery. The symbols which dance through our cronewort-touched dreams pull out the cobwebs of our forgetfulness and assist us in remembering old, unwritten ways of healing and living that attend to the needs of spirit and soul.

Cronewort's choice of home raises the eyebrows of sophisticated folk, for the plant consistently prefers devastated city environs to comfortable country haunts. Walking city streets, one inevitably stumbles across her greensilver leaves flowering out of sidewalk cracks. Fields of cronewort, or hag-weed as I sometimes affectionately call her, sway in abandoned city lots and the thin, grass-enclosed boundaries of highway dividers, where the plant's hardy leaves clean carbon monoxide out of the air, contributing to the health of our lungs and rebalancing the environment. Cronewort was used by Native Americans primarily for its lung-healing capacities, the burned or smoked leaves easing bronchial congestion, its diaphoretic qualities breaking childhood fevers, flus, and colds.

A long-time emblem of wildcrafters, cronewort, like the thirteenth fairy, never fails to show up uninvited on the doorstep of the herbalist devoted to using wild common plants for food and medicine. One student of mine, after her first summer of herbal studies, was surprised by a lone mugwort which appeared in the window box of her second-story Manhattan apartment. Though cronewort generally avoids rural areas, an herbalist friend I know who lives on 100 acres in upstate New York found a single plant by almost stumbling over its four-foot tall stalk which had leapt up by the steps to her porch.

Cronewort's own growth cycle resembles the shifting form of the goddess from maiden to mother to crone. The young cronewort unravels its feathery, gray-green leaves and casts a magical shimmer over a muddy, early-March ground, where islands of snow lay sooty and unmelted in the earth's hollows. In spring, the entire surface and underside of each leaf seems to be dipped in a lime-green down and moon silver glow which beckons bare feet to wade through its mesmerizing sheen. These young leaves, added to salad or dried and smoked, revive energy by stirring the heart into the cackling, chuckling laughter often indulged in only by young children or very old people.

I remember a Halloween women's weekend where we were intent upon visioning; we made homemade cronewort noodles with the spear-shaped, aerial leaves of the fall plant we had gathered during the day. We drank infused cronewort and before bed, we smoked dried cronewort leaves, asking the spirit of the ancient wise woman to send us visions. While most of us did indeed have magical dreams, our cronewort experiment had some unforeseen side effects. While sitting by New York's

Hudson River, attempting to sing the solemn rounds of an old pagan death and rebirth song, each time I looked into the face of the woman with whom I was partnered, the two of us burst into fits of uncontrollable laughter, till we were clutching our bellies and tears ran down our faces.

While the rhythm of our singing was broken, cronewort had brought us the gift of vitality through letting go to chaos and the unexpected. Cronewort is a wonderful ally for those who feel themselves to be too restrained; coming to know this plant inevitably causes unpredictable behavior that heals rather than hurts, coaxing our bodies and attitudes out of stagnation, helping us remember merriment of spirit. Those whom this grandmother weed has befriended are distinguished by the mischievous spark in their eyes.

As mugwort matures, its elongating leaves divide like those of the maple tree; much like a human hand, the sun-exposed side of the leaf grows darkly green and toughens; the weed's underbelly however, remains silver and soft from the swan-white down which covers it. The dual nature of the leave's appearance reminds me of my own temperament: one face of my self often turned out to the sunlit world, and another belonging forever to the dark, my ear tuned to the swish of melodies emanating from the black of night and illumined by the full face of the moon.

Indeed, known to many as an herb of magic, cronewort allows us to live in several worlds at once, expanding and nourishing the habit of drawing our gaze before us to that which is visible, and behind us to that which is invisible. Regular use of cronewort in tea or extract strengthens our ability to absorb intuitive information as we preserve an aspect of sharpness in our interaction with the complex, topside world. This skill is often attained only by those who are of substantial age, but the canes of the elder cronewort, whose seed-heavy stalks bend toward the ground like the spine of an old, wizened woman, assist all in developing this art.

Burning the smoke of cronewort has a similar effect; for this purpose, a small bundle of fresh cronewort gathered at the full moon is wound round and round with silk embroidery thread and hung upside down to dry. When the leaves are crisp, you may use the bundle in personal ritual, igniting the tip and letting the smoke waft through the room. Some say the flowering leaves gathered on June's full moon are best for visioning purposes; I myself prefer to use flowering tops which have been harvested in the fall.

Like a true wise elder, cronewort knows that a grounded, vital body is as precious as our visionary abilities, and so *Artemisia vulgaris* tones our organs so that we will become sturdy as well as wise old crones. Cronewort leaves are a rich source of vitamin B complex, vitamin C expressed as ascorbic acid, and carotenes expressed as vitamin A. Cronewort abounds in minerals such as calcium, potassium, phosphorus, and iron. A vinegar made from the leaves of this artemisia will strengthen the entire digestive tract, improving appetite, normalizing bile production, and supporting and restoring the supple strength of the small and large intestine. Sluggish digestion disappears with regular draughts of the infusion, the walls of the digestive tract responding quickly to the stimulating, camphorlike oils, slight astringency, and vitamin and mineral richness of its leaves.

Like its much more potent cousin wormwood (*Artemisia absinthium*), cronewort extract or infusion uses a firm, deft hand to eliminate worms and parasites from the digestive tract. Cronewort's gentle but clearly anthelmintic quality kills worms and simultaneously tones the weakened walls of the gastrointestinal tract. An infusion of the herb, drunk several times a day for an entire moon cycle—particularly over the full moon as this is when worms propagate—will help the intestines release the worms. A single drop or two of wormwood extract added to the infusion will speed their expulsion. A dropperful of cronewort extract of the leaf or root, taken similarly, is also effective and can be used for children's pinworms.

In my own city garden, very nearly forested with mugwort, I observe the golden staves of cronewort bow toward the ground, remaining unbroken as winter winds rustle the empty husks of their beadlike seed capsules. Dead, each stalk is still sturdy enough to bear even the weight of snow on its slender, withered frame. This habit reminds me of cronewort's skill in keeping the bones of menopausal women dense and flexible. Prepared as a simple vinegar from leaves at any point in its growth cycle, cronewort's calcium richness tends to women's physical strength, keeping bones from becoming porous and preventing osteoporosis as the menopausal body seeks assimilable sources of calcium.

Cronewort is first and foremost a woman's weed, its affinity for the moon and female cycles reflected in the silver palm of its leaves. A hormonally balancing herb, cronewort may be used through the waxing or waning periods of the moon (from new to full or full to new) to urge a woman's womb in remembering its cyclical connection to the moon, slowly restoring her menstrual rhythm to its natural cadence. Used in this manner, cronewort teaches young women a grandmother's knowing and pride in the gift of our menstruation. The bitter principles in cronewort strengthen the liver, assisting it in releasing those hormones into the bloodstream which shape the tempo of the menstrual cycle. Cronewort's nervine qualities surround the sensitivity women often feel as we bleed with a protective energy, soothing headache and insomnia. Cronewort infusion eases nervous twitches, shaking, nervousness, and quaking of the muscles when sipped hot as an infusion several times a day for a period of at least three weeks.

In Japan, cronewort's fierce protective quality is well known by household women, who hang wands of it over the door to keep out evil influences. In western Europe, cronewort was worn by travelers to protect them from fatigue, sunstroke, wild animals, and evil spirits. A crown of its flowering tops was worn on midsummer's eve to call in fairies and to assist one in visioning the future. Cronewort tea is used by modern witches to bathe magic mirrors and crystal balls.

Used with motherwort *(Leonurus cardiaca)* and chickweed *(Stellaria media)*, cronewort extract slowly dissolves fluid-filled, ovarian cysts. Cronewort alone is used for dissolving dermoid cysts, which are made of hair, teeth, and nails. Some women have experienced dramatic reduction of ovarian cysts within a single month's time. Others have used the herbs over the period of a year to slowly and steadily shrink these lumps. While cronewort's hormonal wisdom works to dissolve the cyst, sipping the tea often leads a woman to remember the sacredness of her womb, instructing her through dreams and intuitions to take solitary time as the nutrient-rich lining of the womb eases out of her body.

As we defy the negative cultural messages around menstruation and honor this tidal vessel of creation nestled in the pelvic area, the frequency and duration of many women's reproductive ills lessens. Frequent sips of hot mugwort tea or infusion are excellent for relieving menstrual cramps while drawing out the cronish visionary powers of the menstruating woman in her dreams. A poultice of the warm leaves on the belly also eases menstrual pain. Midwives, assisting mothers in childbirth, use the steam of cronewort as an analgesic to ease the pain of birthing mothers and to help bring down afterbirth. Sitz baths of the infusion help the woman's body release the trauma of birth from the muscular and nervous system.

Cronewort eases the pain of pelvic surgery, where it can be used until the acute situation has subsided. Cronewort roots, in conjunction with other herbs, have been used as an emmenagogue, and are mentioned by Hippocrates as being successful for this purpose. I like to keep an infused oil of mature cronewort leaves on hand for rubbing into the skin of any woman whose pelvic area is distressed due to any reproductive challenge. I also infuse the young and mature leaves in olive oil for cooking and salads; the infused oil has an earthy flavor and adds a bit of digestive zest to one's meals.

Cronewort's pain-relieving and warming effect is well known in China where, for thousands of years and still today, cigars of mugwort are rolled and ignited, the smoke burned near kidney points to relieve lower back pain, kidney distress, and cold. The application of mugwort smoke near the skin is called moxibustion, the rolled cigars of the downy plant known as moxa sticks. Administered in the Chinese fashion or sipped as infusion, the effects of mugwort can be felt in the urinary tract, where the plant's complex mineral richness restores the symmetry of electrolytes which might be unbalanced by the diuretic properties of the herb. Used as a vinegar, cronewort eases stress on the kidneys, dissolves kidney stones, and dissipates water retention.

Cronewort's analgesic abilities are drawn out of the plant into either an oil or water base; a bath of cronewort infusion eases rheumatic and joint pain, and cronewort oil spread gently over arthritically afflicted and pained joint areas greatly revives damaged or inflamed nerves and brings warmth into the joint capsule as it dulls pain. Like the knowing hands of the wise woman, cronewort oil seeps deeply into muscles and joints, permeating the cells with sensation and relief. Steaming bowls of boiled cronewort are often placed between the feet of a squatting woman in labor, to ease the deep internal cramping and draw down the afterbirth.

I often add cronewort oil to violet or Saint-John's-wort oil, the cronewort helping these other oils travel deeply to the root of pain in muscular tissue or joint capsules. Cronewort makes a potent, deep green, belly oil which can be rubbed externally over the womb and ovaries to relieve cramps and help dissolve cysts. Early-seventeenth-century herbalist Culpeper recommends cronewort as an ointment to "take away wens and hard knots, and kernels in the throat . . . three drachms of the powder of the dried leaves taken in wine, is a speedy and certain help for sciatica."

Cronewort also possesses antifungal abilities, and can be used on athlete's foot or fungal patches. The sensitivity to fungus experienced by those with candida albicans (thrush) and the HIV virus are assisted by regular ingestion of cronewort infusion. The fresh juice of cronewort has been used to stop the itch of poison ivy, to repel mosquitoes, and was traditionally used as a special remedy for overdose of opium. While few use opium today, this information indicates to me that cronewort might be a suitable ally for those recovering from heroin addiction.

There is one last skill cronewort possesses, an invisible one familiar to those who seek out the nonphysical, unscientifically proven medicine powers of the plants. The fresh juice of *Artemisia vulgaris*, released by rolling and crushing the leaves, flowers, or seed capsules between thumb and forefinger and then annointing the brow in a moonwise direction, opens the third eye, the psychic visioning center. Cronewort assists those who are touched by its strong scent in deepening one's connection to the world of dreams.

✑ Mugwort Dream Pillow

mugwort leaves
hops flowers
lavender blossoms
mint leaves (just a pinch)
1–2 cups of flax seeds
1 yard of silk or soft, natural material such as flannel
a small zipper

For this recipe, you may play with some of the herbs, always making cronewort the primary herb, as it is the strongest for enhancing dreaming. I put in lavender, for the scent soothes my nervous system, just a wee bit of hops because it is sedative and strong smelling, and a touch of mint to enhance clarity in my dreaming. You may want to do some research into the properties of herbs for dream pillows. For example, lemon balm, linden, and chamomile are popular additions to the pillows of children, for these herbs calm them. Eyebright can be added if making an eye pillow, or elder blossoms, for soothing the eyes.

The amount of herbs will vary according to the size pillow you make. I cut two rectangular pieces of silk in a muted color, long and wide enough to stretch across my eyes for use as an eye pillow. I first sew two long ends together (inside out), follow around the short corner, and up the other long side. At the last end, I sew in the zipper. While I am sewing, I pay careful attention to what I am thinking, since I want the pillow to have a particular effect. I sometimes sing as I work, making up verses to the crone, or simple rhymes which focus my intent on remembering my dreams.

In a bowl, pour in the cup or two of flax seeds. Hold the dried mugwort in your hands and rub it over the bowl, releasing some of the oils as you drop the leaves into the flax seeds. Then add a small amount of hops (no need to crush them, the smell is already powerful), crushed lavender blossoms, and the mint. The pillow should feel full, but with some room for the flax seeds to slide around inside it.

✑ CRONEWORT NOODLES

This recipe comes courtesy of Susun Weed, the herbalist who midwifed the wisewoman tradition of herbal healing. Many thanks to her for her courage in remembering and voicing our common, non-sensical women's lineage as herbalists and healers.

> *1 egg*
> *½ tsp salt*
> *2 tbs of powdered cronewort*
> *or 3 tbs chopped dried or fresh leaves*
> *1 ½ cups of wheat flour*

If you are making the powdered cronewort, use a mortar and pestle to powder by hand. Beat the egg and salt until thoroughly mixed. Stir in the cronewort and flour. Keep adding flour until you have a stiff dough. Knead for five minutes, adding flour as necessary. Roll very thin, cover with a damp towel, and leave the kitchen, resting for twenty minutes or so. Then cut the sheet into strips and dry a bit before boiling.

✑ CRONEWORT VINEGAR

I find this vinegar so tasty that I make it from young leaves, mature leaves, and flowering tops from March through November. Follow the directions for making vinegars in the January chapter.

✑ INFUSED CRONEWORT OIL

I like to make oil from the maturing leaves before they flower, and though I haven't tried it, I bet oil prepared with the bending canes of cronewort gone to seed would be helpful for the arthritic pains of the elderly. Oil from cronewort gathered on the new moon might help quiet menstrual pains; on the waning moon, to help dissolve cysts.

cold-pressed olive oil
fresh cronewort leaves
jar
labels

If you plan to use the cronewort oil for cooking, use a high-quality olive oil. If you are planning on using the oil on the skin, you may experiment with grapeseed oil or stay with the olive oil. Follow the directions for making oil in the March chapter. After six weeks, decant and apply generously to affected areas.

℮ CRONEWORT HOUSE PROTECTION CHARM

three wands of flowering cronewort
colored embroidery thread
doorway

You may play with the colors you would like to use for binding the wands together. If you worship a particular deity who protects you, use the colors of that god or goddess. I like to use red, black, and white, the colors of the triple goddess. Some traditions use red ribbon to dispel the evil eye, others use light blue for protection. Bind the bottom end of the three wands together, imagining, with each turn of the thread, that you are wrapping your home in a protective field. Drape the bundle over the doorway for a full year, and then replace.

DREAMING

The wise spinner who plaits the future and understands the proper time to give death is called to us as we sip cups of cronewort tea during this season of the dark. While I cannot scientifically explain to you which volatile oils in the plant stimulate dream activity, cronewort undeniably causes a shift in the strength and content of one's dream life. For those who have difficulty remembering dreams, cronewort will assist one's recall; for those whose already court their dreams, cronewort spurs the archetypal figure I call the dreamkeeper to summon ancient symbols from deep, forgotten psychic locales and present them to the dreamer as a means of inspiration and guidance.

The dreams one has while using cronewort as an ally often touch the dreamer on a gut level, magnifying the internal voice of instinct and acting as a catalyst for change. One may begin to ask specific questions of the dreamkeeper during the dark time of the year which, through serious intent and the conscious building of a dialogue between one's self and the dreamkeeper, opens the gate to a magical realm of dreaming populated with animals, magical figures, portents, and visions of ancient ways.

To delve fully into a discussion of dreaming is beyond the scope of this book. However, I do consider dreams mystical pathways, usually buried and hidden beneath fallen leaves, stones, and tree roots in the psyche which the dreamkeeper, upon asking, sweeps away, allowing dreams to be used as a sacred bridge between the conscious and unconscious mind. Dream matter offers, in a personally symbolic way, directions for our growth and protection, often presenting the true dynamics of life situations our conscious mind may be unwilling or unable to see and accept. Dreams alert us to soul attrition and offer solutions which renew possibility; we may be visited by dead relatives who assuage our grief and replenish our faith. We may be whispered warnings when the ego is about to make a choice detrimental to the life of the soul. Often, when we ask from the heart, we are given clear indications of directions we need to follow that lead us, eventually or immediately, toward increase in wisdom, soulfulness, and humanity.

Hecate, the keeper of the crossroads, is an old triple goddess who, in her death form, rules the season of the dark. She represents the energy which knows how to anchor the power which exists at the meeting place of three roads; she knows how to be still, her cauldron before her, and stir the frothing contents of her blackened cooking pot until the time of action comes. The months between Halloween and Winter Solstice teach us to practice Hecate's art of remaining solid when our roads are crossing; when we are consciously giving death to aspects of our selves and our lives, when what we have known is dying away, and when we are faced with the need or desire to take a turn in our paths. The raven that sits on Hecate's shoulder represents the part of ourselves adept at flying off and retrieving information we can then add to our cooking pots until the time for movement occurs.

Dreams act as the raven to the one within us which sits, waits, and stirs the pot of change during the season of inaction and invisibility. Dreams fetch symbols and objects from the scope of vision available to flying creatures and present them to us. Our work is to learn how to interpret the meaning of these gifts and to integrate these conclusions into our understanding of ourselves. Dreams let us know both where we have diverged from the cycles of life, death, and rebirth and what needs to be done to keep our loyalty to this rhythm close to the heart.

REMEMBERING

I have come to deeply trust the material given to me in my dreams; I consider my dreams to be messengers from the soul, supportive of my living a life touched by the enormous sacredness of the elements. When my mind turns back to times in my life when I felt unalive, stuck at the bottom of a dark well in which skylight had dwindled to the size of a pinprick miles and miles away, I see that my connection to the awe and magic of life had been severed. At these times I was often given deeply magical dreams. Single words and potent images rang loudly to awaken my drowsing faith and acted as the rungs on a ladder fashioned of live trees, infused with the pulse of life. My hands around each rung of the ladder were touched by the spirit of life once again and gave me the elemental strength necessary to pull myself out of the well of despair.

Within that well, my eyes experienced a blindness in which I was unable to see what was needed to help myself. These moments of forgetfulness have given me the understanding of what leads people to harm either themselves or that which is innocent and natural outside of themselves. It is when we lose our mindfulness of the miracle of life that we become dangerously capable of killing. I have witnessed this cycle over and over again in my own community garden, where some people divide plants into levels of importance based on their looks, dismissing nutritive weeds as garden "pests," and believing themselves to be in control of nature rather than in partnership with it.

Several years ago on a summer day I went to the garden, basket and knife in hand, to gather cronewort from a corner patch in my plot which I was tending for the making of vinegar. My heart was filled with the serenity I often feel while on my way to gather plants. When I reached my plot however, I was dumbstruck, for rather than being greeted by the tall greensilver stalks of artemisia, there was a gaping hole in the corner of the plot. Someone had pulled virtually all the cronewort out of my garden. After staring unbelievingly into the upturned earth scattered with bits of silver leaves, I sank to the ground and began to cry. The violence of the act toward the earth struck me in my heart. A woman gardening near me came by, looked at the damage, and muttered something which dismissed the gravity of the situation. I just cried harder and sat there until I had no tears left.

My grief emptied, I asked the cronewort what to do. She very simply said "there is no killing me." Wild weed that she is, the cronewort did grow back. And I learned that for myself, rather than diminish the injustice of inhumane acts, I want to become like the crone, who represents the mature force within us that is willing to see things as they are, and determine what medicine needs to be applied. Regular ingestion of cronewort builds this fierceness within us and allows us to bear unpopularity in order to remain close to what we know to be true.

Drinking cronewort, we become like the old woman whose blind eyes belie the vast reservoir of vision awake within her other senses. We begin to use another form of seeing, using our hands to caress our environment, identifying by feel those things, ideas, and people which carry life, meaning, and magic. I believe cronewort is called "forgetful" because she is medicine for those who have forgotten the beauty of all the plant represents; the hag of the plant world, cronewort assists us in remembering our simple, common wildness, our connection with the moon and magic, our experience of sacred menstruation, and our partnership with the atmosphere.

Perhaps most important of all, sipping cronewort infusion, or even deeply smelling the oils within the fresh leaves, awakens eyes within us capable of seeing the immanent magic of the earth we walk upon. Our ability to see the earth in this way is crucial for creating culture which sustains and supports the rhythms of nature, governed by the threads of life, death, and rebirth.

For the whole month of November, offer yourself to your dreams. Keep a journal by your bed, or a tape recorder. Before bed, either drink a cup of mugwort tea, smoke a small cigarette or pipeful of cronewort, or rub some cronewort oil in between your brows. You can also light some dried cronewort leaves in a small bowl and inhale the smoke. You may decide to craft or purchase a small dream pillow filled with cronewort and other herbs (directions on page 17) to keep next to your pillow. Sitting up in bed and following your breath, quiet the mind and practice turning the eyes inward and seeking the place within you where the dreamkeeper lives. He or she may be in the heart or the belly; she may live in the back of your head. Ask the dreamkeeper a specific question if you have one, or simply ask that you remember your dreams.

Keep a notebook within reach, so that when you awaken you needn't make large motor movements to find it. Write your dream down in the present tense, beginning with "I am. . . ." Writing in the present will help you stay in the realm of the dream. With regular practice, you will be able to write your dreams down quickly and without completely awakening yourself, so that you can return to sleep. Practice for the entire month, recording the date of your dreams, the weather outside, the position of the moon, and if you are a menstruating woman, where you are in your menstrual cycle. Over time, you may begin to notice several patterns emerging; there may be figures in your dreams who reappear, places you return to again and again. During the day, you can give some thought to interpreting your dreams. I have found though, that simply by staying faithful to recording my dreams, another aspect of knowing surfaces within me which understands the meaning of my dreams in a nonanalytical fashion.

One of the greatest gifts of touching the world of one's dreams is that it is uniquely personal and therefore has one's deepest interests at heart. The act of remembering dreams nurtures our relationship with ourselves, enriches our sense of mystery and continuously helps us be surprised by previously unmet aspects of our own nature. Struggling to interpret our dreams is like learning a language; while we may feel frustrated to begin with, ultimately knowing this language opens up worlds.

Practicing dreamwork in the month of November, we have the blessing of the spirits and the magical world upon our efforts, and we discover a deep inner richness that dwells in the land of the dark, replacing our fear of going within with the peaceful satisfaction of meeting the magic that lives within us; we find that though the trees are bare, our inner lives are teeming with fertility.

DECEMBER

❧

Centering, Illuminating, Giving

—and it is possible a great energy is moving near me.
I have faith in nights.

—Rainer Maria Rilke

I DISTINCTLY REMEMBER the feel of December's darkness in the Brooklyn of my childhood, for in the heart of winter my reluctant eyelids opened not to the wan light of an early winter morning, but to a room brimming with darkness and suffused with a penetrating draft. My ten-year-old mind devoted itself to inventing ways I could dress for school without having to leave the cocoon of heat generated by my own body. I was shocked by the reality of venturing out into a dark world accompanied by the hum and false glow of street lamps and unattended by the rustlings of squirrels, who heeded the rhythm of the dark by remaining in their oak-leaf nests.

I instituted my own emergency measures in response to this night which persisted into the beginning of my morning. Before bed, I laid my clothes for the following day by the radiator so that they would be infused with a heat that instantly warmed my skin. Sleeping in footed pajamas and wrapped in my father's terrycloth robe, when my alarm rang I leapt to the radiator and pressed my back against its slats. Clenching my teeth, I bore the moment of peeling off my nightclothes, shivering as I drew on tights, blouse, and skirt, warm and stiff as toast. Layer by layer I shrouded my body in this clothing that had soaked up a night's worth of refined heat.

By the time I stepped out into the street, I was well protected against this unwelcome winter night which visited my day, though I grumbled miserably as I walked through the halos of my own breath, trudging the two blocks to school. Eyes cast down, I kept my thoughts of the cold at bay by counting the miniature ponds of ice that reflected the light of each street lamp arcing among tree branches out into the center of the road. If there was snow, I took to the road from the sidewalk, my eyes riveted upon imprints left by the tread of snow tires. Through thinly slit eyes I imagined these marks as a hieroglyphic language which had been left by those who had perished in the high, endless banks of snow and piercing cold as they journeyed, hungry and complaining bitterly, to school.

As a teenage Jewish girl, Friday's sunset meant the segregation of the common workday from the holy Sabbath by the lighting of a pair of candles at the exact moment of nightfall. During the week, as my study day was long, I often watched the waning of the day and the seeping in of night through the dipping fog of frost that sheathed the windowpanes of lab class. The clear winter sky, spilling its light below the horizon, became blue-black, the glow of sunset fused with a darkening mantle that threw the unadorned arms of the local elms and maples into shadow. My consciousness felt torn as I struggled to focus on the glaring unnatural lights of the schoolroom and logical subject matter, for my skin trembled, attentive and thrilled as it returned again and again to the magical and nurturant field created by the arrival of the sloping night.

At the end of the school day, I pulled from my locker the thermal underwear, fleece-lined boots, earmuffs, hat, scarf, and hood which comprised my winter gear and wrapped myself to brave the tundra of Avenue J. The warren of life between Sixteenth Street and Eighth Street was a terrain so familiar to me I did not need eyes to see my way home. The shops stood firm as trees; shoe store, card shop, optician, florist, and meat market had all been rooted to their locations for decades. As I walked with chin tucked in my scarf, my shoulders instinctively knew when I passed Gottlieb's, the kosher bakery where red and white string hung down from a metal hive suspended from the ceiling. Women served from behind the counter, their upper arms soft as the loaves of bread they placed in waxed-paper bags, expertly winding the striped string around and around boxes in which they gingerly placed cakes pulled off the plastic discs in the window display. Pearls of water, condensed by the mating of heat and cold, dripped down the glass panes and hid the confections from the view of those on the street.

Face buried like a young swan against the wind, I knew when I passed the Key Food grocery by the salt that crushed under my boot heels and left lace-thin white lines in the leather of my snow boots, and by the pillars of boxes I slipped between as though darting through a maze. Turning right after the storefront sign, I pushed my weight into an old wooden door whose glass was opaque with mist and protected by chicken wire. Once inside this space, my whole being relaxed into the deep heat that generated from an enormous tin drum filled with boiling water. An old man and woman, swathed in what seemed like homespun burlap rather than clothing, took turns skimming a huge wire spoon across the roiling surface of the water, filled underneath with rings of dough that would soon be bagels.

Placing my eight cents on the counter, I asked if anything was hot. "Hot, Hot," the man sang, "everyone always wants them hot." He smiled and I endured the tweaking of my nose. The lenses of my glasses fogged. Using a set of tongs the length of his arm, he opened the oven and reached deep into its back. My head reeled and my mouth watered from the comforting scent of yeast and onions. "Special for you," he said, dropping not one but two bagels into a brown paper bag. Reaching in, I kept my gloves on to handle the oven-fresh bagel that gave off steam as I tore it in two. I kept the other bagel in a bag I placed behind the zipper of my jacket, right by my heart, to keep me warm for the rest of the walk home.

Avenue J, from Sixteenth Street to Coney Island Avenue, was lit by both street lamps and the indoor fixtures of many stores. However, once I passed the Dime Savings Bank and crossed the wide avenue that yawned between the Atlantic Ocean and Prospect Park, I entered a brief landscape that embraced rather than fought the long nights. Even the seasonal Christmas lights draped over the manicured yew bushes gleamed darkly blue as if they had been strung with respect for the special darkness that dwelled in this area. It was in these several blocks that I came to know the holy blackness of which the heart of winter is made, my fear interrupted by the drifts of snow which laid its quilt over lawns, hedgerows, and tree arms. I slowed my pace to an almost stillness by stepping into the lightly sculpted prints hollowed out in the snow by wandering cats.

Pausing to catch the milky pink color of the snow-heavy sky, I listened to the wind speak and let myself be covered in silence. My senses strained to grasp a presence I felt lingered in this place, the way the old goddesses and gods settled down into the sacred groves that had been laid aside to invite in their divine presence. Standing still, my doe-thin ankles braceleted in snow, I felt the darkness comfort me like the rhythmic breathing of a sleeping mother whose oven-warm bed I crawled into.

My active mind filled and emptied with figures I imagined flew through the air under the curtain of the night. Bats, owls, witches, ghosts, cats, and snakes shared this quiet place, riding currents of air and slipping lightly over the snow, perhaps journeying home as I was. I loved them. As I walked through a dark I sensed was crowded with these beings, I felt stripped of isolation and loneliness, accompanied as I was by slow-flapping wings that might be angels or night birds. I came to desire and seek out this immaterial presence that raised the hairs on my nape, quickened my heartbeat, and passed through me like a spirit, for it brought me close to that presence in myself.

CENTERING

On cold nights, often at the tail of the Sabbath, I sat in the small room beside my bedroom. Its six windowpanes groaned from the wind that struck and slithered into the room through the cracked seal between storm window and sill. Wrapped in a blanket and curled on the loveseat, I listened to the branches scratch one another, break off, and plummet downward from the weight of ice; I taught my mind to thrust into the background the noisome hiss of cars hurtling down the parkway and to listen for what barely breathed under these man-made fences against the barren night.

I began to palpate the environment of the dark through what was absent in it: the stark, silent air emptied of bird speech, the branches undisturbed by the scuttle of playing squirrels; a dark so dark no shadows moved within it. I came to understand that the dark was like a wild creature and that to confront it directly was to drive it away. The dark asked to be apprehended by becoming like itself, by finding the place in myself that had no form, which was spacious and black as a hidden cave.

If I had been older, I might have found this task daunting or difficult. As a child, it seemed simple: I closed my eyes and shut out the world, walking into the dark that utterly inhabited my body. This dark seemed parted only by the flesh of my skin from the sweet darkness nesting in the hedgerows of the houses that lined my walk home from school. Bringing inward-seeking eyes into all my interior rooms, I found the dark where loneliness lives, and a dark which soothes its burning despair with a cool, stroking hand. I found a dark that brings sleep, and a dark that invites us to recall the lost skill of night vision wherein all spirits are made visible. I found an enfolding, protective dark force, a dark that spins dreams, and a dark whose vastness struck me speechless. I heard a voice winding out of the dark that propelled me to seek its origin. Tuning my listening and sensitizing my touch, I followed this voice to its creative source, a single note sung or cried by spirits and caught by my seeking heart.

The wind of this creative force gathered like threads within the walls of my physical body, its breath igniting not a light but a husk, for the dark made of its own spirit. This small kernel settled like a pomegranate seed within me, becoming a core to which I could fly or flee when centering was sorely needed. I found in myself a thickly black territory unboundaried by skin and bones that matched the immensity of the cosmos.

ILLUMINATING

In December, the downward, inward, spiral of winter's darkness is arrested by the rebirth of the sun, which slowly unwinds its closed fist of light upon the land, expanding the length of days from solstice onward. These first shafts of light, while still cupped in winter's cold hands, reach out to human spirits weary of the dark with an infant light that softly murmurs of the new life close by. While the return of the light is barely perceptible, honoring its presence gives us strength to endure what remains of winter.

In earth-sensitive cultures, the rebirth of both the dark and the light were understood as kinetically powerful moments of transition; the focused energy released during these crossings of earth, sun, and moon were harnessed through ritual and used to recharge both the human spirit and body. The wheel of the year created by the movement of the planets was seen to pivot only if humans participated in its revolution through dance, song, story, and spiritual calling.

The internal, mysterious personality of the season of long nights tilled a ground fertile for the activities of inner listening and contemplation, out of which new and surprising forms of creation could flow forth come spring. Feelings of boredom and restlessness that accompanied a lengthy spell of darkness may have moved humans to conjure winter celebrations centered on the rekindling of not only light, but human connectedness, joy, and hope.

The rebirth of the sun on the winter solstice causes a tender stirring of the earth out of its own sleep and a yearning in our winter-lulled spirits toward the sense of possibility borne on the rays of the newborn light. Virtually all cultures with a home ground some distance from the equator have woven stories around this rebirth of light, tales I imagine were spun around hearth fires where children and elders huddled for warmth and companionship during the dark season. In these myths, the sun is represented by a divine female or male who is reborn into youthfulness at this time. Old nativity feasts held during December honored the birth of sun gods and goddesses such as Attis, Helia, and Juno Lucina. Today, in Sweden, vestiges of Lucina's worship remain; on Winter Solstice a young girl is chosen as Lussibruden (Lucy Bride), crowned in a headdress of candles, and celebrated in a procession as she-who-rekindles-the-sun.

The Christian church placed Jesus's birthday on December 25 to link Christ's mass with the solstice nativity celebrations that were already in place. Prior to the Roman emperor's acceptance of Christianity, Christmas day was observed by the Romans as Juvenalia, "day of the children," in which folk of all ages were given license to behave as mischievously as youngsters. Children were honored as the seeds of the future through the bestowing of gifts such as bells, hats, socks, and lucky talismans. The entertainment of the day included storytelling, costuming, masquerading, mummery, and theater. It appears that the gay spirit of Juvenalia has persisted into the present Christmas day, at least in the minds of children, who know it as a time to receive gluttonous amounts of attention and have gifts showered upon them.

The Jewish tradition celebrates the miracle and wonder of light in its Hannukah festival. Rather than marking the return of the sun's light, Hannukah commemorates a historical period in which a small clan of Jews, known as the Hasmoneans, defeated the Greek forces who were curtailing the religious freedom of the Jewish community through various edicts and enforced cultural absorption. The victory of the Hasmoneans was followed by a 100-year span of peace.

The miracle of light in the Hebrew tale centers around the menorah, an eight-armed candelabra which was housed in the Jewish temple. Representing the eternal flame of divinity, this lamp was kept lit by a highly refined oil, set apart for the singular task of kindling the menorah. During the struggle between the Hasmoneans and the Greeks, only one undesecrated bottle of oil was found in the temple, enough to keep the eternal flame lit for a single day. Miraculously, the small flask of oil sufficed to keep the menorah's flame burning bright for eight days, until new holy oil could be obtained.

Today, Jews who celebrate the eight-day festival of Hannukah light a candle for each night of the holiday that has passed; by the eighth day, the fully lit menorah is a feast of light for the eyes. It is traditionally kept in the window of one's home, where its flaming beauty can be enjoyed by all. Early Talmudic laws on the lighting of the menorah specify that it be set by an open door, tending the desire that Judaism's unique identity as a religion remain unextinguished, the light of its message reaching out into the world. When I gaze into the eight candles standing side by side in the menorah, I see a symbol of individuality grounded in community. I see the understanding that each human being's way of experiencing holiness is valuable and, when allowed to stand next to others, creates a blazing warmth which indeed, lights the world.

In pagan tradition the idea of eternal return, symbolized in other cultures and religions through the lighting of the flame, is expressed through the ritual use of trees. During the twelve-day midwinter festival, as the solstice light is born, the Holly King, Lord of the Waning Year gives over his sovereignty to the Oak King, Lord of the Waxing Year. The Yule log, hewn of oak, burns for the entire festival, as an emblem of the coming of the new time of growth. The Yule log is kindled from a piece of last year's fire and made to smolder for the entire festival. The cinders of the log are swept together and preserved until the time of the first spring planting, when the ashes are folded into the newly turned earth. This simple ritual demonstrates continuance and renewal, linking what has passed to what is newly born, offering humans the opportunity to relate to the body of the earth with reverence.

Perhaps the most cherished ritual of today's holiday season is the decoration of the evergreen tree. Very few do not respond with a leaping heart to the sight and smell of a resinous pine tree brought indoors and placed in the home, where it becomes a hearth of its own kind. The custom of lighting a living pine tree was brought to England in 1840 by Prince Albert, the German bridegroom of Queen Victoria. The pine tree, which kept its green garb all winter long, acted as a fitting symbol for the promise of new life, a hope necessary during the long winters where darkness fell by midafternoon and a bleak, windswept landscape dominated one's vision for many months at a time, broken only by the presence of these rich, green trees. In this month where evergreens abound and are brought indoors to bedeck hall, sill, and entryway, it is fitting that we discuss the herbal and magical virtues of the evergreen tree which graces our home and keeps our inner flames burning during this transitional point of the winter season.

PINE *(Pinus albus)*

In the 1700s, when Americans were attempting to organize a government, Benjamin Franklin attended native intertribal meetings, for the native peoples of the Northeast had formed (c.1450) an intertribal leadership group called the Iroquois Confederacy, with the singular purpose of maintaining peace. Five tribes came together to learn how to respect one another's traditions and unite rather than war against one another. Several hundred years of peace between these native tribes were enjoyed under the leadership of the confederacy. Some of the principles of government decided upon by the Iroquois Confederacy are believed to be one of the bases of the U.S. Constitution.

The Seneca people (one of the Iroquois tribes) tell that during a time of great bloodshed and strife, a peacemaker appeared among the east-coast tribal nations. The mission of this peacekeeper was to unite the people under the Great Law of Peace. After convincing the tribal leaders to come together, the peacemaker unearthed the "tree of long leaves"— the white pine—and one by one, the tribal leaders threw their weapons into the hole so the groundwater could wash away the blood of death and desire for destruction contained within them. The peacekeeper replanted the tree in its original place and taught the people to meet under its protection, observing that the white pine grew its leaves in clusters of five, each of the five needles representing the five nations of the confederacy.

The peacemaker asked the leaders to note how the branches all joined to one trunk rooted firmly in the earth that reached for the sky. Lastly, the peacemaker placed an eagle atop the pine, to gift the chiefs of the tribes with far vision regarding approaching danger and ability to see the larger picture of life when the details were preventing understanding. This pine was said to have four roots growing out of a center into the north, east, south and west; to return to inner peace, one need only sit beneath the tree and pull back one's energy into the center from all the directions. Thus the white pine came to be called the tree of peace.

The Native Americans looked deeply into the shapes and habits of all beings on the earth to learn of the powers embodied in their very forms. The circular shape of the pine tree and its ability to reach a great age were believed to teach of the endless cyclical wheel of time and the wisdom which comes with travelling many turns around the wheel of the year. According to native wisdom, pine needles, which are wrapped at their base in small packets, were said to remind humans of the strength and sustenance available in unity. The gentle and pliable wood of the pine represents strength in softness.

During my travels in France and Scotland, I had the opportunity to sit in the shade of pine trees that had been left intact for hundreds of years. In contrast to some of the forests of my area, which have been clearcut over and over again, I found fields and glens in these two countries where trees had been given centuries of time and freedom to live and grow. The magic sentience of these trees was undeniably strong. Their trunks stood solid like the torsos of giants, and their branches extended with the complexity and grace that maturity brings.

In one glade in Scotland, I sat beneath a red pine whose girth required three of us to wrap our arms around its waist; its own limbs seemed to arch protectively over the whole forest, gathering all woodland inhabitants in its embrace. The floor beneath the tree was fragrant with foot-long dropped cones; a silent humming that emanated from the tree's trunk and its draping branches lightly struck my eardrums, smoothing out my nerves and filling my head with a thick drowsiness. Beneath this tree, I felt a desire to be quiet for perhaps a hundred years, to lay my head against its trunk and dream. Encompassed in a profound feeling of safety, I curled up for a nap upon the soft earth that dipped between the thick tendrils of the pine's roots, intoxicated by the sweet green fragrance of fallen needles.

Pine is expectorant, demulcent, and diuretic, and has been used primarily by herbalists for those with afflictions of the lungs and disturbances of the bladder and kidneys. The needles of the white pine are rich in vitamin C, and make an excellent vinegar and tea for increasing one's resistance to infection. In the 1800s, plantation slaves boiled white pine needles with molasses as an iron and vitamin C tonic. Infusion of the bark and the needles of the pine regulate mucus secretions in the bronchial passageways, easing tonsilitis, laryngitis, and bronchial troubles. I often decoct a strong infusion of freshly cut pine needles, flavoring it with honey and using it as a gently expectorant cough syrup.

A light antiseptic, white pine can be used externally for skin conditions. Tom Brown, a naturalist raised in the pine barrens of New Jersey, has a deep fondness for pine, as it was the first herb he ever used for food and as a binding agent. Children respond especially well to white pine tea, for it imparts to them an inner sense of peace, as if a loving grandparent were nearby, and the light, tangy flavor of its "long leaves" appeals to the young, often picky palate.

Several years ago I was visiting friends in the Catskills, where I met several young folk. We took a late Saturday afternoon walk in the woods; the day was hot and they were bored with water sports. I led them through the forest, nibbling hemlock tips and tiny violets without saying a word. The three children were clearly enthralled; they had never before seen a human eat from the forest. I led them to a white pine grove I had sat in earlier that morning, and we settled ourselves down on the sweet smelling bed of rust colored needles.

Gathered around a single tree limb, I showed the trio the packet in which the needles were bound, and pointed out the slender white stripe on each of the five needles. When I explained that we could make tea from its needles, they jumped up and grabbed the tree, about to tear off handfuls of pine. Putting up my hand, I explained to them that one of the trees in the grove was the grandmother tree, and that they had to ask permission for gathering first. Halting in their tracks, they stood still, struggling to understand how they could hear a tree communicate. After several minutes, they tiptoed around the small trees in the grove, gently stroking the needles to gather enough for our afternoon tea. Each child thanked the tree in his or her own way.

As we walked back, the girl's hand in mine, she turned around more than once, looking back toward the tree. She asked me if it was possible for humans to fly. As I opened my mouth to think of a response, we were surprised by a flock of wild turkeys, waddling swiftly through the wood. "Anything is possible," I whispered. Upon our return, the children placed the needles on the table. One of them boiled water, another found a large jar, and they all chopped up the leaves and made tea, which they waited until after dinner to taste. The whole process, from our walk to drinking, took about three hours, during which the children were excited by the newness of making tea from a tree. The friend who I was visiting told me that each summer, when new friends come to visit, the children take them to the pine, ask them to guess the grandmother, and teach them how to respectfully gather and make pine needle tea.

The pitch of pine, from old and new wounds to its bark, can be slowly heated and used as an epoxy resin. The resin also draws out splinters and brings boils to a head. The antiseptic quality is quite strong in the resin, and sores, cuts, swellings, and insect bites are eased when thinly coated with it. The thick pitch can be applied to the chest as a plaster for treating pneumonia, its warming and drawing powers being quite strong as it draws blood to the surface of the skin. Extract of the resin in grain alcohol can be used in the springtime to help clear old mucus out of the far reaches of the bronchioles. Soaked in boiled water, the needles can be used in the bath to ease general muscular soreness and sciatic pain, as the circulatory quality warms the cold joints elderly folk often feel in the winter.

I discovered one of my favorite uses of pine during my years as a massage therapist. I chopped up fresh pine needles and infused them in olive oil for six weeks. The result was an incredibly emollient and sweet-smelling oil which deeply soothed the nervous system of many of my clients, gently increased their circulation, and strengthened blood vessels. The slight astringency of the pine makes an oil which rarely spoils; one can also add hemlock tips, cedar tips, or the winter green needles of any of the evergreens for a fragrant winter oil. This oil can also be put in the bath and used to delight the nerves and soothe the joints.

Dr. Edward Bach, the British physician who began to work with flowers for healing mental states, created a flower essence of pine, which he recommended for those who are filled with self-reproach, guilt, and despondency, or who blame themselves for mistakes and are prone to too much self-improvement. The resin of pine can be burned to clear weighty energies from the air, and the smoke is said to repel evil and send it back to its source.

Magically, pine is an emblem of immortality. The Chinese planted it on graves, for the green of its leaves, so strong in wintertime, were believed to be full of chi, the vital force, and could prevent the decay of the dead body while strengthening the spirit of the departed. Branches of pine served a role in purifying areas of outdoor worship, where the branches were used to sweep the forest floor before the performance of seasonal outdoor rituals. In Japan, pine is hung over the doorway to ensure joy to the occupants of the home, and in rural areas, a cross of pine is placed before an unused fireplace to keep evil from entering.

Pine cones have long been considered a symbol of male fertility, particularly in old Dionysian cults, where staffs of fennel were tipped with two pine cones to represent the life-giving force of the male genitalia. The nuts of pine fostered fertility through the sensuality of their creamy texture and smoky flavor as well as the protein richness one received upon ingestion. Pine is a fitting tree to bring indoors as a reminder to keep the Lord of the Waxing Year, who will call fertility to the land by awakening the sleeping underground seeds out of their dormancy, close to our hearts as we inhabit the dark center of the winter season. Both nut and cone have been used magically in fertility charms.

The presence of the fragrant pine in the home fills the very air with the sweetness of life and the anticipation of pleasure; the green vitality of the spring and summer which never leaves the pine reaches out to embrace us in its excitement. In cities, where many humans rarely have woods to walk in, the sight of a tree in the center of the home helps us find that central, calming axis within. Taking time to beautify the tree with handmade ornaments and lights illuminates our creativity.

On a recent solstice, I was at a celebration where we drank hot cider, pierced oranges with cloves, and sewed necklaces of cranberries and corn. When the darkness fell we zipped up our bulky jackets and processed outdoors to a nearby local community garden, where we circled a tree and garlanded it with our decorations. The children then placed red candles in holders with hooks and affixed them to the tree.

Around a live tree of blazing lights, we sang several songs and gave our thanks to the tree. In silence, we watched the lights flicker, their flames sending a welcoming warmth to our limbs stiffened by cold.

As I gazed at the faces of those who clasped hands in a circle, it struck me that we were enacting an old, deeply *right* practice, journeying into the dark with folk of all sizes to the place where the tree was rooted to the ground, circling the emblem of ever-returning life, and leaving it alive as we honored it. To leave the tree undisturbed was an act that recognized our place in the web of life and our role as stewards of the earth. Speaking our gratitude to the tree for its many gifts to us gave all in the circle the great gift of full-heartedness at the darkest time of the year.

ᥱ EVERGREEN WREATH

> *1 long evergreen bough, be it cedar, or any pine/or fallen boughs of*
> *equal size*
> *red berries, such as rosehips or hawthorns (which can still be found*
> *on the trees)*
> *pine cones*
> *acorns or any variety of forest floor seed capsules*

Gather pine branches from a thick tree, remembering to leave the grandmother tree and ask her for permission to harvest. Take pine cones too, being sure to leave a gift for the fairies underneath the tree. To make a wreath, lay out three even segments of boughs, so the needles drape downwards, and weave together as a braid. You may also simply twist the boughs together, the needles all flowing in one direction to represent the wheel of the year. Decorate the finished wreath with the red berries and findings from the forest floor, as well as any other talismans you would like. I often hang a single seed capsule from the top of the wreath so the husk floats in the center of the wheel. Be experimental in your design and you will deeply delight in it. Hang the wreath over the door. When the season is done, gift a tree with your wreath, or burn it in a sweet-smelling bonfire outdoors.

✑ CHRISTMAS/YULE MULLED WINE

christmas tree tips
cloves
cinnamon
allspice
red wine

Combine all of the above and simmer for a long time over low heat. This tonic wine warms the blood while clearing the lungs. Make sure the Christmas tree tips you use have not been sprayed with chemicals.

✑ INFUSED EVERGREEN OIL

fresh pine needles
cedar tips/blue spruce tips/balsam fir tips
olive oil
a jar

I love to combine these three types of evergreen leaves, as the oil they make is absolutely heavenly. Cedar oil is deeply warming and the pine needles bring blood to the surface of the skin, all in a gentle, velvety way. Make as a six week infused oil. Grapeseed oil can be used in place of olive oil.

GIVING

The practice of leaving gifts under the Christmas tree hearkens back to the time where the evergreen tree was worshiped as a symbol of life renewed. Presents were left under the bowing branches of the evergreen in thanks for the ever-returning sustenance gifted to us by the earth. Consciously honoring the miracle of living on an earth that provides for us reminds us that we are blessed with abundance year after year. During the dark time of the year, we may easily forget that we ourselves and the people around us are lights which keep our hearts burning with the flame of love. The practice of gift making and gift giving illuminates the internal shadows which eclipse the full-out blazing of our spirits.

I am fortunate to have a dear friend who has been my teacher in the art of giving. Many years ago, when we were first becoming acquainted, she and her daughter arrived at my birthday party with gifts that were new to me: They made me a card by hand, and created a small book in which they pasted images they had cut out and collaged. All the images in the book reminded them of me; some touched aspects of me I had not yet nurtured in myself, but which they could easily see.

I was deeply moved by the thoughtfulness which had obviously gone into their crafting, and I was also inspired to learn how to give in the same way. My friend is a naturally generous woman who derives great sensual pleasure in cooking and baking as much as she does in making films and taking photographs, which she develops by hand. As an herbalist who makes my own medicines, tonics, creams, and concoctions I appreciate and understand the deep nourishment that comes from handmade work, from allowing one's self to be involved in the organic process of bringing something to fullness and completion.

Deep giving often comes from feeling full within ourselves. However, there are times when, if we feel depleted, making gifts can strengthen our hearts and renew our vitality. A Jewish tale I once read beautifully illustrates this wisdom. In the story a young woman named Eleorah (the name means 'light of god') works night and day weaving prayer shawls out of wind for her people. One spring day, seized by the desire to travel, Eleorah sets out in search of creatures, places, and experiences which expand our sense of life. With each encounter Eleorah's eyes seek awe and kindness, clasping to her heart the warmth and hope she finds.

When Eleorah returns home come fall, she sits at her spinning wheel and threads the exhilaration and joy of these experiences into the prayer shawls and blankets she makes for her community. As the dark nights deepen and the cold intensifies, Eleorah shares her magical blankets and shawls, which wrap the people in the shimmer of spring and summer life, in the abundance and goodwill Eleorah found in her travels and in the quivering joy of humanity which imprinted itself upon her heart.

Like Eleorah, with practice, we can use giving to ignite and sustain a strong flame within ourselves all year long which carries us through the labyrinthine dark of this month and dries up despair as it replenishes our inner warmth. In December, walk out into the world, your mind intent upon seeking signs of life that comfort the soul and enlarge the spirit. You will find these awes and wonders. You will find them in the crescent of the moon and in the crisp black of the winter night. You will find them in the stars of Orion's belt, so sturdily placed in the sky and in the tender hands of the mother buttoning her daughter's coat against the cold. You will find them in the wings of pigeons warming their feathers on the ground, and in the upturned faces of carolers. Breathe them in. Hold them fully in your body, bathing your cells in them, for these miracles replenish and nurture us.

For each difficult and dreadful experience we read of in the newspaper there is an act of deep love which occurs simultaneously. But we must remember to be touched by the brown squirrel gathering dried grass in its paws as it fortifies its nest, for we have grown an armoring of the heart against suffering which has also inured us to these simple miracles.

The more we set up a ground within ourselves which habitually reaches toward the wonders of daily life, the more we can actually turn our gaze toward suffering without shutting down, with a strength that allows us to ascertain what is needed to transform difficult situations. The more gifts of wonder we give ourselves on a daily basis and keep near our hearts, the more we will have to renew ourselves and give to others when our inner lights grow dim, unleashing a brightness which reconnects us to life during this thickly dark, wintry month.

JANUARY

❧

Resting, Being, Listening

LOOKING OUTSIDE MY window on a January evening, I see the dark trunk of a bare oak tree glistening with half-melted icicles, its arms bearing the sweet burden of white snow, a nest of faded oak leaves nestled in the cleft where branch joins trunk. Having drawn its vitality within to protect itself from the cold, the tree slumbers, deathly still in appearance. Keeping its energies dormant, the tree pulls up into her roots from deep in the ground the basic nourishment needed to hold her life force steady until the thaw begins. Snow clings to the earth, warming the soil, its comforting steady fall rendered luminous by the light of the street lamp. The surface of the earth is cold and hard, her inner core a blaze of fire.

Human beings, at our most natural, are no different than the trees or the other creatures of this earth. Our bodies and psyches instinctively resonate with the mood and feel of our environment. Though the daylight begins to lengthen after the Winter Solstice in late December, in January the ground is still frozen solid, the wind so raw it burns our exposed skin with its stinging iciness, the severity of the weather making the nights stretch in our imagination to interminable lengths. During the cold season, creatures respond to the fierce weather by burrowing in their lairs, nests, caves, and holes, sleeping and dreaming. If we allow the wild animals around us to be our teachers, we learn to behave as they do at this time of the year, creating for ourselves a snug habitat conducive to retreat, giving ourselves permission to rest, thereby protecting and maintaining our inner resources.

RESTING

The provision of an interval of rest and retreat are familiar to me from my childhood rearing in an Orthodox Jewish family, where we observed the weekly ritual of Sabbath. The period of time beginning at sundown on Friday and ending an hour after sundown on Saturday was devoted to the practice of resting. As Friday's light began to wane, my mother pulled out the silver tray holding the heavy brass candlesticks and put two new white candles in them, placing the tray on the kitchen counter. As the sun dropped low in the sky, she often raced to complete the cooking of our meal, for it became taboo to continue those labors of daily life which required fire once the sky grew dark.

When the sun slipped below the horizon, Mom opened the drawer where the linens were kept and covered her head with a lace veil my great grandmother had crocheted. As she draped the veil over her hair and around her shoulders my ordinary mother was transformed into a mysterious bride. As I watched at her side, she held her hands over the flames, beckoning three times with her arms, calling in the Queen of the Sabbath, whose dark, fertile energy would invisibly hum in the air around us until that hour after sundown the following day. Hands cupped over her eyes, and my hands now over my eyes, Mom murmured the Hebrew blessing thanking the creator for giving us the task of lighting the Sabbath candles. Dropping our hands from our faces, we gazed into a kitchen touched by the in-dwelling presence of the Sabbath Queen.

For the ensuing twenty-four hours, there was a letting go of work. Time was devoted to sleeping, studying, reading, sharing meals, and sensing within these more meditative activities the presence of the Queen. The enforced leisure of the Sabbath hollowed a space in which one could *be* rather than *do,* and experience the timeless serenity available in just being. Liberated from the distractions of daily chores, one could more easily notice the simple blessings of life. The environment of the

Sabbath created a mysterious vessel, pregnant with possibility, in which vitality could be renewed and new form initiated. It is no surprise then, that this energy was embodied by a female, queenly symbol. Amongst the commandments given to the Jewish people regarding the Sabbath, couples were bidden to make love on this day, for the restful conditions ripened the chances for conception to occur, and a baby conceived on the fertile Sabbath was said to have the Queen as her guardian.

I must confess that as a child, an entire twenty-four hours of nondoing was torturous. By nightfall on Saturday, I was quite ready for the closing ritual. Huddled in the dimly lit kitchen, we held a braided candle aloft to symbolize the entwined energies of life, death, and rebirth. Singing a farewell song to the Sabbath Queen, we inhaled the scent of cloves from an ornamented silver box as a reminder to keep Her sweetness close by all week long. Lastly, we extinguished the candle in a saucer of wine. With the snuffing of the flame and the switching on of electric light, life instantly turned mundane, as if Cinderella had suddenly lost her ballgown and returned to her place by the fire, raking cinders. Weekly I looked forward to the renewal of soul that was the gift of performing these rituals, of watching, sniffing, and handling the candles, the veil, the flame, the cloves, these objects weighted with meaning, each Sabbath.

Scent, symbol, dance, and song which revolve around the rhythms of light and dark, earth, sun, and moon, move us out of linear time into magical time. Weaving our joys and sorrows into this web renders our human experience holy and places it alongside the daily miracles of sunrise and sunset. Glimpsed through the eyes of ritual, the winter season is a sacred, beauteous time that allows us to touch our own holy, interior ground of being. Awaiting the twilight in stillness, we open to the possibility of joining with this moment, of feeling the waxing and waning light with our very bodies, kinetically discovering just how closely knit we are to these wild, natural cycles. Our very bones remember and yearn toward them, for when we align ourselves with the elemental rhythms, we feel fulfilled and connected to an immensely soulful source.

In cultures where people worked the ground for their sustenance, winter was a time when food that had been stored was used for nourishment. On the practical level, food supplies needed to last until the ground thawed enough for plants to grow. So there was a natural respect for winter as a time to simplify one's physical activities, thereby lessening the need for replenishment through the conservation of energy.

In the United States, we live in a culture where most of us purchase rather than grow our own food, and our homes are more often than not heated mechanically rather than by way of a roaring fire. Yet, like the lean oak tree outside my window, in January we instinctively contract against the cold, seeking within rather than without for *how* to nurture ourselves, as if the human body's desire to remain kin to the elemental rhythm of the winter season still guides us. In the hushed mood of this month, we can cultivate a ground of silence in order to hear the quiet whisperings of intuition about how to best comfort and feed ourselves. Like the young, slumbering oak we can weather the winter by sleeping well and preserving our energies, gracefully accepting the gift of winter and the opportunity for simply being that it offers us.

BEING

January's drowsy stillness creates an opportunity for us to give not only our bodies but our minds a rest from planning, worrying about, and negotiating the future. The leanness of the environment, trailed by the coming lush growth of spring, offer us the certainty that inactivity precedes the emergence of new life. In some mysterious way, rest and retreat prepare the earth for its next cycle.

In our activity-focused society, it is difficult to trust this unfamiliar cycle of nondoing. Creative artists, however, understand from personal experience the need to respect this invisible, fallow period, for it is the foundational ground of creation. I have been told that Virginia Woolf, at the start of a new novel, placed a blank sheet of paper in her typewriter and stared into it daily, sometimes for months on end, waiting for an idea to form and take root on the page. Through cultivating the habit of patience with the nondoing aspect of her writing process, she learned to engage with the void as a necessary, receptive part of engendering creativity.

The sparseness of the earth and sky, the sharpness of the cold in January provide a pristine clarity which snaps us into the present moment. The frozen air jars us awake, alerting us to the here and now. Much in the way the Buddhist tradition uses meditation as a means of practicing the art of being, a tender attending to the winter environment can bear similar fruit. In January I use the habitual, daily acts of self-care to frame the present moment of being and to stay within its core. While washing the dishes I follow the course of water back to its source of cloud and am grateful for it; as I turn the dish in my hands I think of the elements which created it: fire, earth, and water. As I cook for myself, I drink in the intertwined scents of grains, vegetables, and spices and am nourished even before I taste a morsel. By firelight, as I write in my journal, I listen to the scratch of my pen against paper, my thoughts settling like snow so the deep and simple stirrings of my being can emerge onto the page.

In January I savor the ordinary: the sound of the kettle, whistling and shaking upon the stove as the water boils, the taste of tea as I sip from a favorite mug, the yeast-sweet aroma of bread I am baking. I write letters by candlelight, read winter poems, and watch my breath puff white clouds into the air. I pause by fences and roof eaves to run my fingers along the toothsharp points of icicles. My eyes settle on the bulky feathercoats of sparrows, gathered in trees still ringed with holiday lights. Indoors, I brush my cats, who spend much time on the window ledge, flicking their tails back and forth at those same plump sparrows. This interior, soulful time falls into the realm of the Lord of the Shadows, who fills the darkened chambers of our beings with a fullness made manifest as our listening and perception grow keen enough to catch the quiet gifts of the dark season.

Attentive to the slower hum of my body's energy, I listen to its signals and heed its messages. Am I tired? Do I need more sleep? More heat? Are my feet warm? Have I caught a draft in my ears, or on the side of my neck? Do I feel peaceful, or agitated? What are my dreams telling me? Though I love the crispness of the air in winter, that my body contracts inwardly in search of heat tells me I need to choose and use those herbs and foods which keep the blood circulating freely, such as ginger, garlic, and thyme.

There is no doubt that January is a difficult month. To rest and reflect, to nourish one's inner self in a culture which places little value upon reflection is a revolutionary act. For some, the darkness and temperature mingle to produce feelings of isolation and despair. Gazing into the flames of hearth fires, which naturally produce warmth and encourage reflection, has been replaced by staring into the light of our TV sets. Settling our eyes on the radiance of even a single tongue of fire renews our sputtering inner flame, reassures us that the sun's warmth will return once again. Herbal potions brewed at this time serve to brighten our internal fire, giving us comfort, nurture, and pleasure as we use them in soups, baths, and teas all winter long.

Often in winter, if I ignore my body's cold weather needs I get sick, usually with some malady that keeps me from speaking. I am reluctantly forced into silence and self-tending, drinking teas which cool and contract inflamed throat tissue, bring down my fever, keep me warm, and lift my spirits. Garden sage and thyme are plants which possess these gifts and thrive in pots in the kitchen as well as out in the garden, making them available fresh all year long for use in cooking as well as medicine. The ability of these plants to thrive outdoors during the winter months is testimony to the strengthening qualities they impart to us, helping us to take winter in stride.

GARDEN SAGE *(Salvia officinalis)*

The Latin name for sage, *Salvia,* means "the healing plant," and its even older root word, *salvus* means healthy and sage. The dictionary definition for the noun *sage* refers to an elderly person who is venerated for his or her experience, judgment, and wisdom. Legend has it that those who eat sage become immortal in wisdom and in years. There is an old monk's statement: "Why should a man die whilst sage grows in his garden?" and an old English rhyme: "He that would live for aye (ever), must eat sage in May." It was believed that the plant would grow and whither in keeping with the rise and fall of its owner's success in business, and that a thriving sage plant was evidence that a strong, wise woman ruled within the doors of that house. Magically, sage is considered a mother protectress plant and is governed by Jupiter, the planet that encourages nourishment, play, expansiveness, and joyful living. Sage has often been used in charms to manifest wishes and attract money.

The gifts of sage affect the brain, the nervous and digestive systems, the joints, the mouth and one's mood and is an especially beneficial herb for women entering the menopausal years. Sage contains high levels of calcium, critical to the strength and health of the bones and teeth, the functioning of the heart and other muscles, the maintenance of metabolism, and the flow of nerve impulses. Consistent use of the tea or vinegar, particularly by women during the menopausal years, will help prevent osteoporosis. Supplying a steady, easily assimilable source of calcium to the body during the hormonally volatile years in which women cannot store calcium is crucial to maintaining bone density.

Sage also relieves joint aches caused by mineral deposits at the joint site. These deposits, often caused by the ingestion of unassimilable forms of calcium, such as calcium supplements, dissolve when the body absorbs the simpler, more bio-available form of calcium it receives directly from the whole plant. I love sprinkling dried sage leaves into soups, for a bit of extra spice in salads, and in salad dressings, to sharpen my senses as well as provide me with nutritional gifts. The mineral richness of garden sage helps men and women age with grace and hardiness, enabling us to endure rough winds and still maintain a spritely humor.

Disinfectant, antiseptic, and astringent, sage is excellent for tightening and healing infected and unhealthy gums and preventing bacterial buildup. Take a fresh leaf and massage your gums with it, or rinse the mouth with tea that has been steeped for about ten minutes. Daily rubbing of the gums with just several sage leaves will heal bleeding and inflammation of the gums, tighten pockets formed by heavily swollen gums, and clear the teeth of plaque.

A group of young students I taught became quite affectionately attached to sage, which they nicknamed "the toothbrush plant," after I demonstrated for them how to rub their gums with the leaf. Each day following that lesson, whenever we passed the "bibilical" garden (which contained three large sage bushes), they insisted we sidetrack behind the walled enclosure so they could brush their teeth.

If you peer closely at a sage leaf, you will notice large pores, which hint at the plant's relationship to the skin. As a facial steam or hot infusion, sage opens up the pores and induces sweating, sweeping away grime while bringing down fevers. Conversely, the drying quality of sage closes the pores and tightens tissues and membranes, relieving children of fever and menopausal women of cold and hot flash sweats. *Salvia's* astringency has made it a well-known herb for drying up the flow of milk in lactating mothers. This same drying ability absorbs excess mucus congesting the throat, lungs, and gastrointestinal tract and reducing the swelling of sores and stings.

Sage's opening qualities extend upward into the brain, where its saponins keep the blood flowing freely, easing headaches and allowing maximum absorption of all nutrients into the bloodstream. Perhaps this herb's popularity in French cooking is due to the presence of carotenes in *Salvia*, which strengthen the liver and prevent digestion-induced headaches. The essential oils in sage encourage the production of digestive enzymes and stomach acids, allaying nausea, indigestion, and gas. When I am drizzling butter over homemade popcorn, I toss in crushed sage leaves to assure easy passage of the oils through my digestive tract. The volatile oil in sage actually strengthens the ability of the digestive tract to absorb rich food.

Breathe in the smoke or steam of garden sage to keep the mind quick, improve memory and transform mental attitude. Simply inhaling the scent of leaves crushed between your fingers will tickle the brain and dispel a sluggish mood. The rejuvenating oils of sage recharge the body with new vitality. I particularly enjoy sage footbaths (see directions at chapter's end) after a long hike in the woods. An infusion of the leaves, applied topically, darkens the hair.

In times past, the older folk carried the responsibility of eldering, of being committed to the community, of speaking for the preservation of resources for generations to come and for keeping hope alive among the people. A sage was one who had lived through many turns of the seasons and had developed the capacities of deep listening, clear reflection, and compassion through the experience of living. All these qualities are essential for the transformation of grief and depression. As we inhale the vapors or smoke of sage, we absorb these strengths, restore our weary spirits, and ease grief.

Garden sage was the first tea I ever prepared from fresh leaves plucked by my own hands. Living in the city, I had joined a community garden near my house and was sharing a plot with a fellow gardener. When the plot was first given to me, I was so bedazzled by the gnarled and twisted torso of the sage bush, by its multi-pored and pungent leaves, gray green-silver color, and smooth, soft feel, that I could not up-root the existing plant in order to claim the garden as my own. Instead, I picked leaves off the plant's uppermost parts, tugging gently to allow the mature leaves to offer themselves and leaving the younger leaves to grow stronger. Wondering what gift I could leave in exchange for the plant giving of her body to me, I pulled off a silver hair from the new cluster sprouting out of my hairline, and placed it at the base of the bush.

At home I placed the leaves in a ceramic mug and poured boiled water over them, letting the water and plant oils merge. As I inhaled the earthy fragrance wafting up in the steam and sipped my first mouthful of tea, I had a fleeting vision of my eastern European ancestors. I saw women dressed in long skirts and babushkas, their thick fingers gathering the plants they needed into their skirts and deftly tying up the hems. Their faces were joyful and their manner secure, perhaps in knowing their food and medicine was provided for, abundantly, by the earth, their true mother.

It is my belief that the plants contain within them the spirit of the land which they originally inhabited. When I sip sage, a native of the Mediterranean coast, I feel the freshness and wildness of that area fill my lungs and refresh my spirit, as if I've walked the shore and been de-lighted and renewed by the sea air.

ᴄ～ FACIAL STEAMS

1 handful of each:
dried sage leaves
dried pink and red rose petals
dried lavender blossoms

dried comfrey leaves
1 qt of water, boiled in a big pot

Facial steams are one of my favorite ways to go inward. You can't get much more internal than putting your head over a steaming pot and covering it with a towel! When the water boils, toss in all the herbs. Let it all boil for a minute or two, then turn off the flame. Have a towel nearby, large enough to cover your head with so you feel like you are in a cave. Duck under and inhale. The sage, lavender, and rose petals are all tightening to the skin and a delight to the nose. The comfrey leaf is moistening, and will give your brain a taste of green and the promise of spring in the dead of winter. When you first go under, the steam will be very hot, and you may only last a short while. Take a break, and head under again. Repeat for as long as you can stand it.

᧕ SAGE BUTTER

1 stick of organic butter, softened to room temperature
fresh or dried sage leaves, to taste (if they are dried, use less, for the
sage oil strengthens this way)

There are two ways to make the butter. If you have fresh leaves, chop them up and whip into the butter. Then you can use the butter as a spread. Otherwise, melt the butter over a low flame and sprinkle in dried or fresh sage leaves. This second method is best for popcorn, the first for slathering on fresh-baked bread. You don't need to use a lot of sage leaves, as they are quite strong. But if you want to, do: you'll become a feisty, resilient elder.

᧕ SAGE VINEGAR

apple cider vinegar, or balsamic vinegar
fresh garden sage leaves
glass jar, preferably with a plastic lid

Fill a jar with fresh sage leaves to the top. Pour the vinegar over the leaves. Press down the sage leaves with a chopstick. Make sure the vinegar comes to the very top of the jar. Cap the jar and put your label on the top. If you are using a jar with a metal lid, place a piece of waxed paper between the lid and the jar, because the vinegar rusts the lid. You can use the waxed backing of labels as a way of recycling. The sage needs to steep for six weeks in the vinegar to allow all the nutrients to move into it. When ready, you can drink the vinegar, a teaspoon a day in water, for one fourth of your daily calcium needs. Or add to soups, mix into your salad dressing: Yum!

℮ SAGE FOOTBATHS

2 ounces of dried garden sage leaves

1 qt water

½-gallon jar

Put the dried sage leaves in the jar. Bring the water to a boil. Pour the boiled water over the sage leaves, filling the jar to the very top. Using an airtight seal and cap. Allow the sage to steep for four hours. This method is called a full-strength infusion. Drain off the liquid into a pot, and re-warm to the desired temperature for your feet. You may dilute this a bit if you like. As you sit with your feet in the basin, sip a cup of sage or thyme tea.

THYME *(Thymus vulgaris)*

The bushlike sage and the diminutive, low-growing thyme thrive well beside one another in the garden and are sturdy siblings in the mint (Labiatae) family. Plants in the mint family, in general, have a beneficial effect on digestion, ease headaches and increase one's energy, can be used to warm and cool the body, and enhance mental clarity, thereby expanding our ability to be in the present moment.

The name *thyme* comes from a Greek word meaning "to fumigate."

Thyme, being antiseptic as well as aromatic, was used as an incense to purify the air and chase insects from the house. It was also used as a house blessing herb and was added to brews which aided one in communing with the deceased. The word *thyme* was also derived from the Greek *thumus*, meaning courage. A sip of thyme cordial had the effect of invigorating the drinker, inspiring him or her to acts of fearlessness. Thyme was an emblem of chivalry and bravery, and women in medieval Europe embroidered a bee hovering over a sprig of thyme on the scarves they presented to their knights.

I tend to pay careful attention to the folklore around plants; often the information derived from *folk,* that is, lay people who used the herbs, is both practical and wise. When I read of thyme as an herb of courage, I am tempted to try out thyme in a situation where I need strongheartedness. If it works, my story becomes part of this folklore, and I pass the information on. When one consciously uses an herb for the purpose of enhancing a particular emotional quality or physical strength, the herb becomes one's *ally.* As you drink, the plant transforms you: its powers become part of your cellular make-up. When thyme strengthens and builds the tissues of the lungs, the lungs themselves can then do what they were created so beautifully to do.

Thyme hugs the ground as it grows, creeping across sun-drenched areas, near ant hills and on heaths. It thrives on rocky ground, where it loves to absorb the reflected heat of stones. Thyme is under the dominion of the sun, the star which rules the heart, circulation, the spine, and the vital force and heat of the body. The sun energy thyme soaks up makes it a fitting herb to call upon in January, where it imparts heat to the body as it is rubbed between the palms into soups, infused and sipped as a tea, and steeped in a most relaxing bath. In Arab countries, thyme is dried, powdered, and mixed with coriander seeds, sesame seeds, and salt to produce za'atar. The za'atar is then mixed with olive oil, spread on bread, and eaten daily.

The beneficial effects of thyme are felt in the digestive tract, lungs, blood, and nervous system. In the digestive tract, thyme eases gas and expels worms. The tea relieves indigestion, inflammation of the liver, and bad breath. In the lungs, thyme is used with plantain (plantago major) to assist those with asthma, pneumonia, and chronic bronchitis. Antispasmodic, thyme stops spasmed coughing and, taken as a steam, helps sinus congestion. Thyme's expectorant and astringent qualities dissolve mucus and clear phlegm from the lungs. Thyme gently dries up the moist coughs of babies, and regular use of the tea will strengthen lungs which have been weakened by coughing, smoking, or infection.

My favorite way to take thyme is as an infused honey. Because the plant survives so well outdoors even in the winter months, I can pick fresh thyme leaves and steep them in honey even in the dead of winter. The aromatic oils of the thyme blend with the antiseptic qualities of the honey to produce a most sweet medicine, which I spread on bread and eat or drizzle into soup stock when I am feeling cold, weak in the lungs, or in need of hardiness. The antiseptic, antibacterial, and biotic quality of thyme strengthens the immune system and makes thyme suitable for poulticing wounds, sores, and external inflammations. A vinegar in which thyme leaves have been steeped for six weeks can be rubbed on the temples to alleviate headache or hangover. Thyme is taken with rosemary to ease migraine headaches.

Thyme is a calming tonic to the nervous system, smoothing out ragged nerves which are the result of overstimulation or inflammation. Prolonged use of it will comfort an anxious stomach; nervous children greatly benefit from thyme baths, as do feverish ones. The heat of thyme, in the bath, will have a diaphoretic effect, bringing on the sweating which breaks fevers.

An herb pillow, (directions on page 17) sewn in a calming color and stuffed with dried thyme can be warmed and placed over the stomach for those with stomach aches or nervousness centered in that area. The thyme pillow protects the sleeper from nightmares and one made with thyme, chamomile, and yarrow will heal those suffering from facial neuralgia. Used for this purpose, the affected person should also drink two cups of thyme tea a day.

Tincture of thyme rubbed externally on affected limbs revives atrophied muscles which have been paralyzed or affected by stroke and strengthens the limbs of children. Drops of essential thyme oil, diluted in olive oil and applied externally, bring blood to the surface of the skin and ease sore muscles, rheumatism, and those working with the effects of multiple sclerosis. The essential oil is antifungal and can be applied similarly to treat ringworm.

In upstate New York, the lilac-colored and maroon flowers of thyme carpet the mossy ground like a soft bed. Lore has it that the Queen of the Fairies lives in the thyme and that the soil where thyme grows in abundance becomes a powerful vortex of energy. Laying on a mound of *Thymus vulgaris,* one will be visited in dreams by the fairy folk. Folklore tells us that thyme was known to bring its wearer vitality and strength as well as enhanced psychic powers. Sacred to Venus, regular draughts of tea open up one's contact with the ancient nature religions. Used in the ritual bath, thyme washes away the sorrows of the past.

I met thyme on November 1, the Day of the Dead, several years ago. I knew nothing about the plant, but noticed that it grew close to the ground, was flowering in the cold, sent up a spicy scent as I stepped on it, and no matter how hard I tugged, her roots held to the earth. I loved the opportunity to guess at the qualities of a plant I had not yet studied, so I sat and listened, hoping to hear some wisdom or insight about the medicinal properties of the plant. What I heard startled and comforted me: thyme said that she kept warm by living close to the ground, which she described as her mother's body, and attributed her lush, ever-spreading growth to staying in touch with her roots. She suggested I do the same.

✐ THYME BATH

> *2 cups dried thyme*
> *2 qts boiling water*

Bring two quarts of water to a boil. Strew in the dried thyme. Cover and steep over a medium flame for ten minutes. Start the bath water. Drain the extract and add to the filled bathtub. Bathe for ten to fifteen minutes. When you emerge from the tub, wrap yourself in a bathrobe and lie down under the covers. Rest for thirty to sixty minutes while you sweat.

The wrapping and resting phase is crucial if you are using the bath to bring down a fever and should be done only once a day. If used for calming or ritual purpose keep a pale blue candle lit as you bathe, and adjust the resting phase as you like.

For the ritual bath, you may use several drops of thyme essential oil instead of preparing an infusion. Drip in a single drop at a time, as the volatile oil is quite strong and a bit goes a long way.

℮ THYME HONEY

1 empty glass jar with a wide lid (use a large jar; you'll want lots of honey)
enough fresh thyme to fill the jar
clover honey (local honey if possible, no preservatives added)

Fill the jar with fresh thyme leaves. If you are gathering leaves in the summer, follow the path of the bees. They pull pollen from the sweetest flowers. Hum as you go, nibble as you gather, and look for fairies. Bring it all back to your workbench, where the jar is waiting. Fill the jar almost to the top with thyme, and pour honey over it. As the honey rises, so will the thyme. Keep a chopstick nearby and keep pressing down the thyme, causing air bubbles to rise. When the bubbles are all popped, fill the jar to the very top with honey and cap. Honey will drip down the sides of the jar, so put a tray under it. Using a self-adhesive label, write "thyme leaves and flowers in honey," marking the current date and the date six weeks from that day. You may dip into the honey during the six weeks if you like; the fairies always do, but replace the honey so the jar remains full.

After the six weeks, the honey will have thinned out and will carry the strong taste of thyme as well as its lung-healing properties. It is not necessary to take out the herb from the honey after the six weeks. Thyme is antiseptic and so is honey; there is no danger of either spoiling, and they can be stored in the cupboard indefinitely.

LISTENING

To me the most precious gift winter brings us is snow. Snow profoundly changes our visual reality and suspends our daily routine. During a recent January blizzard, New York City was declared to be in a state of emergency, but the snowstorm hardly seemed to cause the frantic emotion I associate with crisis situations. Rather, people seemed to slow down, to take a break from business, and enjoy themselves. It was a rare and magical experience to walk the streets without the sounds of buses and cars whizzing by, and to be gently passed by a fellow New Yorker gliding over the snow on a pair of skis.

Blizzards, however, are a rare occurrence on the island of Manhattan, and in our technologically laden era we rarely have or take the opportunity to walk with silence as our companion. In a culture that encourages us to be active and productive in every moment, to be aimless often inspires fear and judgment. It becomes, therefore, a soul-feeding *and* radical act to take a walk through the falling snow, to wander through its twinkling, swirling veil with no other goal than to mingle with our surroundings, to be altered and blessed by the snow as the rest of the environment is altered and blessed.

Snow brings with it a silence that creates the groundwork for listening to occur. Deliberately walking out to meet the snow, it becomes a beloved subject we rest our attention upon, discovering that the white crystals cloaking our shoulders also settle their attention upon us. At first our walking is for ourselves, to restore us to our true place in the natural world. But as our listening comes fully alive, enabling us to take in sounds and textures which add to the richness of our environment, we become connected to all that surrounds us. The matrix of silence which snowfall creates allows a chorus of sounds to emerge into the foreground: a branch breaking from the weight of the snow, the muffled crunch of boots trudging through white earth, and the hush of wind pouring through trees and buildings.

This month, on a snowy evening, make a date to walk with the snow. Dress warmly so that you can spend substantial time out in its world. Before you go outdoors, chop up some fresh ginger root in a saucepan of water. Bring it to a boil and simmer for a while, until you are ready to leave. Then turn off the stove and let the roots continue to steep.

If there is a park nearby, this is the ideal place for a snow-walk, as a tree wears the snow like a jewel. You may want to take a friend with you. If so, make a pact between the two of you to spend your walking time in complete silence, keeping yourselves connected by linking arms. After you have roamed a bit, find a special spot where you can pause for a moment. Closing your eyes, take several breaths in and out, inhaling the silence of the snow into your body. Then cock your ears, listening for the sound snow makes at the moment it touches the already fallen snow. Expand your listening to include all that moves around you.

When your senses are filled with snowy beauty, return indoors and change out of your wet clothes. Gently heat the ginger root tea and pour yourself a mug, letting the delicious liquid warm you to the end of your toes. If your feet are cold, you can pour some of the tea into a tub of hot water and soak your feet in it. Turn down all the electric lights in the room and sit by the window, gazing at the snowfall from your cozy indoor lair.

In this quieted state of mind understanding deepens; we come to recognize in the sound of the wind the rush of our own blood coursing through our veins. We see that this very snow which temporarily changes our routine will eventually melt and become the water which fills our streams, rivers, and reservoirs and feeds our thirst. This snow will moisten the earth and prepare spring to return in her green glory.

As our capacity to listen grows, we are able to recognize that the snow is a being also, with its own need for silence and comfort, with its own passions and dreams. In the wisdom that arises out of the quiet, we see that the snow comes to us out of its own need to give, to bring restoration, to be known by humans and other creatures as a sentient being who yearns, as we do, for connection. Our efforts to fully engage with the snow through silence and listening reclaims its holiness as we rest and learn to simply be through each icy white, January night.

FEBRUARY

❧

Quickening

COME FEBRUARY, THE blushing light of dawn insinuates itself more boldly across the landscape of the day, and as our eyes absorb the increasing brightness of the sun, subtle tremors rise from within us to meet its broadening glow. Though the air still contains winter's crisp bite, all creatures begin to shiver, and our trembling is caused not purely by the cold but by an excitement that begins to blossom down deep in the gut, an instinctive knowing response to the coming renewal heralded by the expanding light.

It is as if, quite unexpectedly, we who were lost or wandering enchanted through underground caves in our polar imaginations feel a ray of sunlight touch that sliver of exposed skin at our wrists, where the coat sleeve ends and our gloves begin. The unexpected rush of penetrating warmth halts us in our tracks, jolting us upright, eyes open and alert. In a single instant we are drawn out of the womb of the dark, and we begin a spiraling journey upward and outward toward this tremulous feeling that desires us and pulls us to itself like a hungry lover.

And what is the name of this force that makes its way into the body rhythm of the animals and wakens them from months of dreaming, that pierces the ruminating dark with the light touch of the sensuous dawn, that makes us toss restless, when we had been so cozy in our warm beds, for winter's end? The name of this power is desire. The desire of life itself for new life, the unavoidable yearning of the dark for its bride of light. And this desire has a heat, and this heat causes a stirring, and the stirring causes a quickening, which causes a flickering flame to wake the bodies of all creatures with a tongue that speaks wordlessly of mating.

The message of desire that rises with the cry of the bluejays into the widening belly of the dawn sky is carried in the warm, inmost center of the still-cold wind for all to sniff with quivering nostrils. Though we may bury ourselves, like the groundhog, under cover of the frozen earth, desire will still come for us. We have no choice. All are summoned, all are made to shudder from the magnetism of this scent conjured by the crone as she begins to draw away the cape of winter. Keeper of all cycles, the wise old woman who teaches us to weather the time of decrease with contemplation and dreaming now rouses us slowly and gently from hibernation, bidding us by the thawing light to make love with life once again.

In ancient Rome, the rising heat of the mating dance was marked through the festival of Lupercalia, which celebrated the ripening sexuality that permeates nature during February. The very name of the month translates as "the month of fever," and Lupercalia refers to the mythical she-wolf, Lupa, who suckled the abandoned twins Romulus and Remus, Romulus eventually becoming the founder of Rome. Wolves came to be seen as a sacred emblem of the Earth Goddess in her nurturant, breeding aspect, their behavior watched carefully as a kind of oracle or omen. February's increasing light triggered the wolves to couple and signaled observant priests and priestesses to descend into the grotto of the she-wolf and join in rites of lovemaking practiced to ensure a fertile spring.

On the Celtic wheel of the year, the eve of February 2 marks the feast of Brigid, a generative goddess who was associated with the fruits of the earth and the fire of the hearth. A shrine to her was located in Kildare, where a holy well and eternal healing fire was kept by priestesses of this goddess. Because the country folk were slow to change customs of worship, as Christianity spread through Europe the Celtic Brigid was subsumed by the church into its canon of fictitious and actual saints. The mother goddess and her mythos became enlaced with the story of a human woman named Bridget, who was deemed a saint in the Christian tradition for her abundant good works.

The mortal Bridget lived in Ireland during the fifth century, where she decided at a young age to consecrate her life to religion. As there were no religious houses for women, she made her abode in the trunk of a giant oak tree which had formerly been the site of the mother goddess Brigid's sacred grove. Bridget most likely sensed the charge that had built up around the tree from years of ritual, and made her home in an already sanctified place.

Other women were drawn to Bridget, and she eventually founded a sisterhood devoted to teaching and charity that became the first convent. Bridget's cloister became a great center of learning, where women and men thrived under her inspiring leadership. One of the services her abbey offered was to provide help, advice, and education to the local peasants. Bridget also established a school of metalwork that crafted exquisite utilitarian objects in its fiery forge. Bridget traveled all over Ireland, establishing convents modeled after her own; she was much loved and later canonized by the church.

Bridget's emphasis on education, creativity, and giving embodied the aspects of the mother goddess worshiped by the earlier Celts; these qualities may have made the countryside people receptive to Christianity, for her expression of it was so similar to the personality of the mother goddess they already honored. The goddess Brigid eventually came to be called Bride, the matron of poetry, smithcraft, and healing. The priestesses (and later nuns) of Brigid were known as brides, for they vowed themselves to this goddess as one would in a marriage bond and kept a sacred fire burning for her at all times.

Most likely the fire that was kept kindled at Brigid's shrine was the huge fire of a forge, which burned meltingly hot in preparation for smithcraft, the domain of this goddess. The unfailing attentiveness to the fire by the nine priestesses of Brigid (and later Hestia and Vesta) underscores fire's fragile aspect, the potential of this extremely important source of our light and heat to be extinguished if we neglect to feed it with new kindling. The brides remind us to tend to all that the fire represents: our creative lives, the passions that keep us vital and joyful, our sexuality, the love and care that kindles our hearths and invites intimacy, and the power of loving nurturance to magically resuscitate that which, left unattended, had seemed to die.

Even as the tender flame of sun and light begins to send its presence over the earth, come February, my wild spirit inevitably becomes shriveled from that sweep of time, too long, where my eyes seek and find only buildings, with their angles and lines, sharp corners, and narrow slits of sky. By February, so many months have lapsed with only the barest moments of green flitting across my vision, my inner ember has all but turned to cold, grey ash.

Now that this phenomenon has happened so many times, over the years, I have come to know what I need: to pass my eyes, either in memory or in the flesh, over rolling hills where the wind impresses itself upon the grasses, making the earth move like an undulating coverlet hung to dry in the breeze and sun. Sometimes it is green, bending reeds I see, sometimes a golden cloak covering the curving mounds which rise beside one another like the many-breasted goddesses of old. Even the coarse brown winter fur that beards the earth revives my spirit and soothes my eyes which have grown weary of the city's harsh topography.

Grasses are the earth's hair. In humans, our head and body hair, and also the cilia, internal hairlike processes which line certain passageways of the body, serve a variety of purposes. The first function of hair is to protect, by catching in its shaft all that it deems must not enter the body. Grass, as it drapes across the earth, restrains unwanted energies in its fringed curtain. Human hair protects the scalp from injury, from the strong rays of the sun, and acts as a barrier between the fragile, innocent aspects of ourselves and the outside world. Tall grasses keep the ground cool in summer, so that nutrients in the soil remain moist and continue to feed all that is growing. In fairy tales, the long locks or whiskers of a wise person often keep treasures hidden until, at a dramatically precise moment, they are revealed; grass also contains this sheltering aspect, harboring in its thicket vulnerable creatures such as the small wren or newborn swallow, who are often hunted by predators.

Surrounding the root of the hair shaft is the hair follicle, which in turn is circled by many root hair plexuses. The plexuses, or nerve endings, are extraordinarily sensitive to touch and make possible the other function of hair as a highly acute receptor of sensation. On a physical level, these nerve endings around the hair allow us to feel touch; but psychically, arousal of these neural tips alert us to the presence of palpable energy, and in the deeply developed manner of the blind, to read the intention of that which we are sensing to bring pleasure, danger, or a wide range of messages.

If one believes, as I do, that the earth is a living body, then it follows that the grasses of the earth make her a deeply sentient being, and that whenever we come across stretches of wild grass, we have found regions of heightened energy and tender sensitivity in both the earth beneath these grasses, and in the substance of the wild grasses themselves. Grains, which are the seeds of the wild grasses, carry within their tiny husks the physical nutrients that sustain us. The more invisible gifts of the wild grasses to humans and other animals are: to protect us when we are vulnerable, and to restore and to strengthen us so that we can shelter ourselves and harbor others in times of vulnerability. Both the minerals in and the erotic nature of grain and grass which we ingest give us heightened sensual abilities that make us profoundly alive and therefore able to love and deeply experience life on this beloved earth.

Grains contain water, carbohydrates, fats, proteins, vitamins, minerals, and fiber, almost all the foundational nutrients essential for life in all animals. Their genetic treasures, housed and protected in husks and hulls, give grains a resiliency which allows them to be stored and transported without damage or spoilage. Grains have the capacity to reproduce themselves a thousandfold; grains which have been found in ancient tombs retain enough life force to sprout and reproduce after thousands of years. It is no wonder then, that grains were considered holy manifestations of the fruitful force of nature which was worshiped in early harvesting cultures in the form of a goddess.

Demeter, a Greek grain deity of the Cretan people, was the goddess of agriculture, responsible for the cultivation of the soil. She was depicted holding a sheaf of barley, a handful of poppies, and one snake in each hand. Her fecundity was celebrated through the Eleusinian mystery rites each year at harvest time. While the articles she clasped have come to symbolically represent the mysteries of creation, death, and regeneration, the ingestion of fermented grain, poppy nectar, and snake venom were used ritually to open psychic doorways through which one's consciousness could descend and glimpse the actual face of these hidden processes.

It is said that through Demeter's creative force, seven grains spilled from the fertile lap of this ancient mother goddess at around 12,000 B.C. Wheat, rye, barley, millet, rice, corn, and oats, therefore, all possess divine chromosomes that become part of our bodies when we ingest them. Once we know the origin of these grasses, eating grains becomes a sacred matter. Today, the grains of these stalks, protected to varying degrees by husks, hulls, and pods, are cultivated extensively by humans for food.

The last of Demeter's offspring, the wild grass of oats, carries the compassionate temperament which must have sparked the abundant creatrix to give us the gift of the grain, for oats love to nourish humans deeply, offering themselves abundantly and willingly as food and medicine for our nerve endings, endocrine glands, reproductive organs, and skin. Oat grass and oats hone our senses so that by simply closing our eyes, we can hear the wind's long hiss like a snake through the high grasses, be stirred to life in our loins and made ready for spring once again.

OATSTRAW *(Avena sativa)*

From their original home in the Mediterranean and near east, oats have spread all over the world, blanketing the great plains of many continents. Unlike other grains, which are wrapped in a single husk and spiral upward toward the sun, oat plants house their seeds in a double husk that drapes downward from a podlike hull. Oats thrive in the chill, wet sea climates of England, Scotland, northern Europe, and northwest America, where the fresh moist sea air fattens the grain and the harsh winds and sudden storms have, of necessity, given rise to a plant adaptable and fierce enough to withstand these weather conditions. In the Middle Ages, as people received the benefits of increased mental endurance and physical strength a regular diet of *Avena sativa* brings, oats replaced millet as the staple grain of the people. Oats arrived in North America with the Puritans.

Oats and oatstraw (the grass, leaf, flower and grain of the oat) provide the body with calcium, iron, phosphorus, the vitamin B complex, potassium, magnesium, vitamins A and C, fiber, and protein. The nutrient-rich and emollient gifts contained in the oats are released in the form of a milky substance which thickens as one stirs the cooking grain. Come June, the milk of the oat rises up the stem, causing the pods to swell; one nick of the pod with a fingernail and the milk drips out of its purse. The milky, moist film of oats lubricates everything it touches, moistening and protecting the digestive tract and the intestinal wall.

The surprisingly abundant nutrient content and easily digestible form of oats gives this grain a gently powerful nature enormously supportive of children, elders, and convalescents recovering from immune-depleting conditions. Oats love to be combined with slippery elm bark *(Ulmus fulva)*, the nutritious inner bark of the elm tree; the thinly curled and shredded ribbons of slippery elm dissolve into a thick jelly when stirred into boiled water. A porridge of these two make a healing gruel for those suffering from weak digestion, such as colicky newborns or people recovering from chemotherapy treatment.

Although oats have seven times the quantity of fat as rice, they are composed of chemical combinations that protect the heart, balance cholesterol, and assist circulation. In addition to cooking oats as a breakfast food, oatstraw can be prepared and drunk as an infusion to reap these healing treasures. The water-based infusion, golden in color and sweetly mild to the palate, is a cooling lubricant and eases thirsty folk of all ages while keeping the body moist as the earth that lies beneath her growing grass. While oatstraw has a direct effect on the nervous and endocrine system, its enormously rich vitamin and mineral content has a transformative effect upon the deep immune system, gradually changing those who sip the infusion and eat the grain into individuals with physical, mental, and emotional hardiness.

Oatstraw builds strong bones and teeth, stabilizes sugar levels in the blood, and improves blood flow by elasticizing veins and arteries. The calcium and silica in oats and oatstraw improve bone density and glandular efficiency and build inner calm and centering. Consistent use of oats improves concentration and also expands sensitivity to joyful stimuli; the balanced nutrient content of oats replaces mental fogginess with acute mental clarity and increases physical and mental coordination.

A powerful nerve tonic, oatstraw has an uncanny ability to steady easily shocked nerves, calming overstimulated nerve endings as it supports and replenishes depleted adrenal glands. Its calcium and magnesium richness act like the sure hands of a mother upon her fearful child, soothing nerves and emotions that are standing on end, when a single touch or sound is enough to send a human running for the hills.

I consider oat baths and oatstraw infusions necessary measures when healing nervous and emotional breakdown, convulsions, and collapse caused by personal calamity or war. Oatstraw revives numbed nerves, rebalances overwrought nerves, and rewires the nervous system with a patience, wisdom, and understanding sorely lacking in our current systems of healing. I am reminded of the fairy-tale task of separating poppy seeds from a huge mound of dirt in a single evening. Oatstraw possesses this kind of perseverance.

Oat-hull stuffed pillows and mattresses are ideal for those who suffer from postwar nightmares or any posttraumatic stress, allowing individuals to sleep soundly and release the stress of the body into the hulls. For those who are not plagued by suffering, the jostling of oat hulls in the pillow lulls one into dreams of *Avena*'s dwelling places, which are the wide open spaces where the wind and oatgrass make a spine tingling music that calls the snakes out onto the rocks to listen and fills the air with the earth's own sighs of pleasure.

The optimum purpose of the nervous system is to open one's senses to energies coming to us from a vast range of sources; some of these sources, such as moonlight, for example, or the rhythmic crashing of waves on the sand, are stimuli our body welcomes. In our society, where inorganic sounds surround us at all times, our nervous systems tend to become irritated, and our nerve energy shuts down, curtailing our ability to drink in the deeply soul-feeding energies simultaneously occurring and available in the natural world. Regular use of oatstraw infusion restores our ability to receive subtle and expansive energies. A friend's mom, who had lost the capacity to taste and smell her food, began to drink oatstraw. After sipping the infusion daily for a year, she suddenly realized that her sense of taste and smell had returned so gradually she had not noticed. She was once again able to take pleasure in her eating.

In our culture, we often turn to alcohol, nicotine, and drugs to give us fortitude or escape during tumultuous, unbearable situations, particularly because our society hides the commonness of these states and insists that we be "happy" when for many, the actual daily environment humans must live and move in is deeply wounding to the soul. Oatstraw restores nutrients depleted by these other placebos and slowly repairs the broken web of spirit.

Oatstraw also gives us an inner fortitude that allows us to become less unbalanced by the stressful stimuli we encounter on a daily basis. As such, it is an excellent ally for those withdrawing from caffeine, alcohol, tobacco, or drug consumption; it heightens our sensitivity and restores our ability to feel, so that we require little to be moved. At the same time, oatstraw also strengthens the nerves, countering the vulnerability people often feel when they are in the process of releasing their attachment to substances. Often these substances have served as a shield against pain and anxiety and it is unwise to remove them unless a new way of protecting oneself is simultaneously being woven into one's psychic patterning. Oatstraw slowly provides this protective field by strengthening our core of calmness.

Oats and oatstraw are remedies for stress that takes the form of chronic headaches, insomnia, and itchy skin conditions. Severe hair loss, often a sign of trauma of some sort, responds well to oatstraw infusion, especially when combined with the hair-rejuvenating skill of stinging nettle and rosemary oil. Oatstraw encourages sound sleep, allowing the body to reap the energy offered by its nutrients as one rests from a fatiguing day. By strengthening the adrenal glands, vitamin- and mineral-rich oats steadily reverse the fatigue symptomatic of conditions such as Epstein-Barr and AIDS. Oats strengthen the depleted new mother, and provide energy to those who have been weakened by fever. A gentle food, oats can be eaten by those with weak digestion.

Oatstraw is a versatile ally for women journeying through the menopausal passageway, consistent draughts of the infusion reducing night sweats and calming the depression and hysteria that sometimes pass though the body during the menopausal years. Oatstraw eases the intensity of hot flashes, reducing their frequency as the oats restore the vitamins and minerals depleted during the hot flash. Oat baths cool the itchy, burning vulva menopausal women sometimes experience, and keep the vaginal tissues well lubricated. Oats combined with slippery elm moisten the dry mouth that accompanies the vast hormonal shift of menopause, and women report that regular use of oats revives their sexual energy as they enter the crone years. The high calcium and magnesium content of this grain ensures strong and pliant bones for the menopausal woman, the maximum benefits of the nutrients in oats received if one also tempers the intake of alcohol, sugar, caffeine, and tobacco.

Oatstraw stabilizes blood-sugar levels, lessening the frequency and duration of the premenstrual and menopausal emotional swings of rage, depression, hysteria, and irritability women often feel in a culture which values constant productivity and stimulation over the more inward and outward pulse of human rhythm. Solitude and a creative outlet for strong feeling states, accompanied by several cups a day of oatstraw infusion (or a daily bowl of oats) help build emotional steadiness. The vitamin B complex in oatstraw nourishes strong nerves and increases one's ability to perceive psychic and physical energy currents.

Oatstraw's milkiness and mineral richness moistens the glands, particularly the reproductive and sexual glands. By restoring nerves to fully functioning capacity as it lubricates one's internal passageways, oats increase libido. Horses fed on a diet of oats often become "highly spirited." The virility attained through regular consumption of oats stems from the grass's affect on the nervous system; the nerves become so restored to optimal function that one cannot help but reach out to touch and fully receive the pleasure of being touched.

Osteoporosis occurs amongst the women in my family, and so I drink oatstraw on a regular basis for the high amounts of calcium, silica, and magnesium the plant contains. When my own mother began menopause, I was a budding herbalist, and had just discovered that oatstraw slowly and deeply rebalances the endocrine system. I recommended oatstraw to my mom for her menopausal journey, and also because she has had lifelong glandular challenges. My mom enjoyed the light, sweet taste of the tea. She grew so fond of her oatstraw infusion that when I came over to visit, she was a bit reluctant to offer me a cup. Mom was also beginning to experience sweats and flashes, and the oatstraw gave her instantaneous relief in these areas.

However, there were some other interesting side effects to Mom's use of avena; these effects have earned oatstraw not only fame but notoriety. A bloom came back into my mom's face. She began to sport a maidenish red blush on each cheek even in winter time. Her friends of old asked me what I had given her, because she had began to laugh again, and to be outrageous "like she was before your parents got married." My mom even admitted to an adolescent lustiness she found was overcoming her in the months since she had been steadily drinking the herb. My father joked "What did you put in that brew?" After seven years of sipping oatstraw on a regular basis, with no other alterations in her diet, my mom reported that the doctor had found no decrease in her bone density since the onset of her menopausal years.

The saponins in oats nourish the adrenals, pancreas, and liver, and reduce cholesterol and the risk of heart disease, while improving the function of the circulatory system. The heart rate slows, palpitations are reduced, and the flow of blood is steady and smooth. Oats support the heart muscles and the urinary organs. Hot compresses of oatstraw applied to painful areas following a kidney stone attack will bring quick relief from the pain. Diabetics and hypoglycemics also benefit from the sugar balancing skill of oats.

The oatstraw bath is an unforgettable experience. Full baths of oats or oatstraw (recipe below) soak away emotional stress, physical pain in the joints, uterus, bladder, and bones, and ease intestinal spasms and the distress of pelvic inflammatory disease. Dip a cloth into the milky bath and wash away years of stress from the face and eyes; oats contain a natural antioxidant which prevents the fat in the grain from going rancid and keeps one's skin youthfully glowing. Or better yet, make a gentle exfoliant scrub of rolled oats (recipe below) and rub away the mask of anxiety covering your amorous self.

Oat baths send moisture deep into the skin, soothing children and adults itchy from chicken pox, psoriasis, or eczema, and relieve exhaustion while lubricating all the orifices and surfaces of the body. Oat baths carry away the dryness of winter and bring forth the promise of a galloping, lusty spring. Immersing my body in the hot milk of oats, I feel like Demeter myself, and often come back in touch with my own ability to nurture myself through the divine, nurturant strength of the milk-giving oat goddess.

℮ OAT BATH (1)

a large pot
several cups of steel cut oats
water

Line the bottom of a large soup pot with steel cut oats. Fill the entire pot with water and bring to a boil. Shifting to medium heat, cook the oats for several hours. A thick film will cover the top of the water; this film is especially emollient and eases itchiness and scaliness. Put it aside in a separate bowl and place on the driest part of your body. Strain the oats through a wire-meshed colander lined with cheesecloth, and take the bowl of hot milk and add to your bath. Burn dried lavender blossoms in a bowl for extra soothing. Shut the door and soak for at least twenty minutes, covering every inch of your body with the milky water.

The milk of the oats, released in this manner, is an unsurpassable moisturizer for those whose faces and hands endure strong winds or long periods of time in water. The recipe is a must for those who live near the ocean. My friend's husband, a boatbuilder whose hands begin to crack from sea salt, loves to soak them in oat milk prepared in this fashion.

℮ OAT BATH (2)

½ gallon jar
2 ounces oatstraw or dried milky tops of oats
water

Prepare an infusion of oatstraw, allowing it to sit for four hours. Add to a hot bath, and soak. This bath is rejuvenative as well as relaxing, and works well for giving one that extra bit of energy needed to complete the last phase of a long project.

℮ DEMETER'S BEAUTIFYING OAT GRAIN SCRUB

2 cups rolled oats
½ ounce to 1 ounce lavender buds or rose petals
2 tsp of ground almonds
2 tsp white or red clay (optional)
a dash of seaweed (optional)
a blender or mortar and pestle

The almonds supply natural oils as the oats gently rub away dead skin; if your skin is oily, you may want to use more clay and fewer almonds. The lavender, however, is astringent as well as pungent and balances the presence of the oil-giving almonds.

Place all the ingredients in the blender or mortar and blend until all the oats are ground up. When ready to use, place some of the grains in your palm and add water, rubbing into the face. You can also wet the grains and keep the jar in your refrigerator, applying the grains as a mask.

℮ OATMEAL FACE BATH

rolled oats
washcloth
rubber band
string

Place several ounces of oats in a washcloth. Tie the rubber band around the neck of the washcloth and suspend it by string to the hot running water flowing into your bath.

When you are in the tub, squeeze the washcloth against your face. The deeply emollient milk of the oats will run out onto your skin, leaving you with the glow one often possesses after lovemaking. You can also squeeze the milk in the washcloth into your winter dry scalp, or onto areas of eczema or psoriasis or on any rashes, particular in sensitive areas of the body.

℮   OATMEAL COOKIES

> *1 cup rolled oats*
> *1 cup almonds*
> *1/2 cup vegetable oil*
> *1/2 cup maple syrup*
> *apricot preserves*

Blend the oats and almonds in a blender. Pour into a mixing bowl, adding the maple syrup and oil. Form the wet dough into cookies that fit in your cupped palm and place on a cookie sheet. Then press your thumb into the center of each cookie, adding a small dollop of apricot preserves (or any other flavor preserve) into the hollow you have made. Bake at 350° for ten minutes. Let cookies cool before serving.

QUICKENING

When a woman conceives, she often intuits the presence of new life in her womb, though she may confirm her pregnancy through the absence of her monthly flow of lifeblood. As the fertilized egg develops, there is a particular point when motion of the fetus begins and its activity is felt by the woman. This stage of gestation, where beneath the taut skin of the woman's growing belly she feels a moving being, is called quickening and the stirring of new life in the month of February follows a similar growth pattern. While our environment is still likely to be pelted by snow and permeated by frost, beneath this apparent quiescence a restlessness begins to pervade all life. Like the mother who presses a cheek to her child's forehead to determine the presence or absence of fever, if we close our eyes and tenderly stretch a hand along the ground, we will discern a subtle change in the temperature of the earth's skin, or a pulse will rise from through our palms that quietly whispers of spring's coming.

I detect the presence of spring as a scent hidden in the cloak of the wind. As I make effort to fill my lungs more deeply than I am accustomed to in the cold, a subtle warmth strokes my sinuses as the breath passes through. This undertone carries the coming thaw in it, rousing in my memory the time when mounds of snow will dissolve and cast a glistening over the ground as they melt; when the aroma of the soil will once again waft up toward the sun that has awakened it, filling all that has been lying dormant and unborn in the folds of the earth with the desire to rise.

But it is not yet time for full awakening. February is a time of promise, when we must trust in the power and certainty of regeneration though our eyes see no exterior signs of birth. Like the newly pregnant woman, we keep the news of this seed secret, containing and protecting the flicker of stirring life like a hand cupped round a flame we are shielding from the wind. And this is as it should be, for now is the time of anticipation, where we prepare ourselves, with the deep attentiveness of a bride or groom, to meet the beloved called life, who will soon come in the guise of spring to slake our thirst and satisfy our desires.

By faithfully tending the flame, the priestesses of Brigid, and later of Hestia and Vesta, were beseeching a divine force to dwell in their midst, filling the environment in which they breathed and moved with a constant sense of divine presence. Likewise, as we encourage and feed this nascent warmth that presages the death of winter, we join with the sun's warmth that slowly penetrates the drowsing seeds and roots that lie beneath the hard ground in initiating the cycle of calling back the green. Holding the flame of our desires close to earth we gain the attention of the sleeping life below its surface.

Though new life is most alive in our imagination this month, February is the time to nourish the seed of our desires through prayer, attention, and ritual. As the season of contemplation and inactivity draws to a close, we begin to call to that within us which yearns for light, for newness, for movement, though we are still embedded in the frozen ground and dark shawl of winter.

It is the tradition of many cultures to prepare for the coming green by divesting one's self in an active manner of that which is worn. In Sweden, as a symbolic gesture of readiness, on the eve of February 2 folk peel wax off of every candlelabra and candlestick in the house, gathering up all the half-burned candles and melting the old wicks and nubs in a huge outdoor bonfire. We can prepare our home similarly for the transition into spring by taking down old boughs from Winter Solstice and Christmas, clearing the house of all dead leaves and dried flowers that have lost their vibrancy and burning them outside in a fire-resistant vessel. Place into the vessel any articles you sense are holding a stagnant energy.

After the home is lightened, clear yourself ritually of the cold season's sluggishness by immersing your body into a ritual bath. Brewing an oatstraw infusion, light some candles in the bathroom, draw the water, and pour in the tea. Fill a bowl or jug with cool water and place it on the sink. Lower yourself into the tub and soak, letting *Avena* soothe your nerves and wash away winter weariness. When you have completed your bath, wrap yourself in a warm robe and stand before the mirror.

In the glowing candlelight, look into your eyes as you would into those of a loved one. Keeping your gaze soft and steady, name all the qualities of beauty within yourself. When you are done, stand quietly before the flame for a full minute. Then, move to the sink where you have set aside the flask of water. In the Jewish custom of handwashing, one pours water from a jug over one fist at a time, alternating fists and letting the water flow into the sink. As you wash your hands in this manner, name all that is worn out in your life, which needs to return to the earth and sea for renewal.

After purification we turn our attention to beautification. Change into something silky and sensual. Fill the room with candles and light them, one by one, bringing your face close to each flame to feel its warmth. Sit by the candle you feel has the most warmth and light emanating from it and take some time to enjoy the blaze of light. Cupping your hands around the flame, feel your hands fill with light and warmth. Then bring your palms to the ground, asking that the light return to warm the earth and awaken the green, that this same fiery force ignite your passions. Warming your hands once again around the flame, name aloud that which your heart would most desire at this time in your life. Walk to each flame in the room and repeat the gestures.

When you are done, extinguish all the candles and sit for a moment in the dark, seeing your wish incubating in the heart of the fire and gathering flesh in the black tail of the dormant season. For the rest of the month, allow the elements to quicken your desires as you watch the light of dawn grow stronger each day, savor the chase- and hiding-dance of mating creatures and revel in the flutter of your awakening limbs that anticipate the coming of spring.

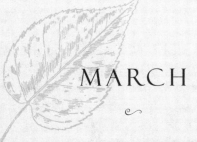

MARCH

Awakening, Beginning

*—to me, a tree is more beautiful than a cathedral. The tree is the
kingdom of god on earth. A tree is the pure land.*

—*Thich Nhat Hanh*

BY MARCH, THE snow-haired Crone, midwife of death, rest, and inward journeying, wraps the veil of winter around herself and begins her retreat to a hidden place. Like a child called home for dinner who scurries to fit in one more hour of play, the last days of winter often unleash unforgettable storms, loosed by the Crone onto the land, till our bodies ache with longing for spring. The gusting weather offers all creatures a last chance to burrow in the heartland of creativity carved out by the snow, to rest in the silence and slow pace of the Yule season.

I have always been struck by the fact that winter seems to ebb in response to a call. In my bones I know that winter herself has a resting place which renews her as we have been renewed by her. When I was a child I wondered where winter lived during the seasons beside her own. Entranced by the way snow dressed the trees, I spent hours at my window following the curve of snow drifts caught in the crooks of branches and between the iron shafts of fence posts, until my imagination conjured another home in a far, undiscovered corner of the great, round earth.

I envisioned winter's quarters as a large, crystalline igloo nestled in the snowy north pole, the outer walls of the dwelling completely studded with icicles. Here, the old woman of winter summered with the north wind, the snow queen, and a variety of wild creatures. When the time was right, she was summoned by the cry of a great snowy owl out of her lair to bring winter's deep, regenerating sleep to all beings, drawing her white coverlet over all.

My childhood quest for winter's secret seasonal hide-out led me, as an adult, to daily observation of the activities of trees, animals, and birds in search of signs that winter's back was turning. One early March day, the air was unusually mild, heavily laden with dew that pearled into droplets that hung off the trees. In the course of a single hour, winter sent out a wind which froze the water so the intricate shapes of every tree branch were traced in ice and the droplets suspended in mid-fall off the swinging chain posts bordering the grass. The weight of the ice, followed by a sudden snowfall of eight inches challenged the limbs to use their strength and flexibility to bear the weight of the frozen water.

While walking down the street, hat pulled low over my ears and chin tucked into my neck, I stumbled into a deeply bowing tree branch that very nearly whipped me across the cheek. Startled, I looked up into the face of my assailant and gasped: the tip of the branch had already begun its springtime growth, sprouting a heart-shaped, furry red, finger-long bud which was now utterly framed in ice.

The image brought me the understanding that the two seasons begin to mesh their energies and that winter slowly *becomes* spring. The tender, early growth of new life in March is strengthened by repeated exposure to winter's conditions. Spring is fattened on the challenge offered by winter's storms and protected by the quiet and solitude woven by late winter's white covering. Something wondrous and vigorous is created in the dark fecundity of cold earth that is revealed as the Crone and her consort, the Lord of the Waning Year, retire. Out of the wintry plunge of the tree's energy into its roots to find life, comes the rising sap of the trees, comes the swelling of buds. As the dying winter hurtles storms behind its back, spring surges upward toward the light. And we, out of the descent into our roots and dark, hidden places, break the ground of our own being renewed and ready to offer ourselves, again, to the world.

AWAKENING

In March the earth receives the melting ice into her body, exposing a terrain with patches of yellowed grass surrounding tiny islands of snow. The bald, muddy soil, rich with water, sinks beneath each footstep that leans upon it, but this mucky dirt hastens the emergence of tender, green tree shoots, of down-covered baby weeds and bulbs planted in the fall. The yearning for newness born of the incessant cold that tossed our restless bodies in February is now satisfied as the dance of change begins in earnest and our eyes, ears, nostrils, and skin are deluged with signs of the returning spring.

To me the force of awakening is most voluptuously embodied by the bursting of buds out of the sleeping branches of myriad trees gracing city streets, country roads, and woodland areas. Indeed, budding time passes so swiftly that *we* must be awake, fully engaging our senses in order to deeply breathe in the excitement of spring's rebirth. There is so much to be learned about our own origins and potential through the thrusting fertility of spring's arrival. As we deliberately attend to the emergence of the buds, we witness the early phases of the spiral of creation, which are often so subtle and fleeting that we would miss them were we not focusing our attention there. Closely watching a bud swell and open on a single tree over a period of several days or weeks can give us a deep and simple understanding about how the web of creation is woven.

We see the tree give birth to a small, delicate, tightly enclosed shape. Gazing deeply at a tender bud, something inside of us knows that other treasures are contained, unborn, within this shape. The mother in the tree, who knows this also, raises the tiny form up to the light and warmth of the sun, our closest star. The sun enters the bud and awakens these other potent elements which have been sleeping inside the form. At the right time, the tree and the sun, the water and the air all call out of the bud the tiny leaves which were inside it, waiting to be infused and nourished by these cosmic powers.

Observing the budding time stirs that in our psyches which knows how to pull up our energies from our internal root system and shape those energies into a unique form. The tree reminds us to offer our infant creations to the earth, water, fire, and air; to steep our fledgling ideas in these cosmic energies so that they may be deepened and unfold in the harmony and power of the earth's rhythms. In this manner, we can create works of beauty which swell and retreat in consonance with the earth's cycles, containing the instinctive pattern of blossom and decay.

Trees are one of nature's greatest gifts to us. They give their bodies to us for furniture, fabric, and rubber, provide coolness through their shade and warmth through the burning of their limbs. Their fruits and nuts feed us and their inner barks, leaves, and branches are herbal medicine. Alive and dead, their trunks are home to larvae, fungi, and a sweeping array of forest creatures.

Earth-honoring cultures all over the world were awake to the vital role of the trees in assuring our well-being and clearly related to the trees as sacred beings. In western and eastern Europe, in particular, trees were worshiped, venerated, and protected for their unique medicine powers. They were considered to be numinous beings whose spirits could be invoked for assistance, and angered to destruction by ill-treatment. Amongst the native North Americans, trees possessed specific emotional qualities such as honesty, strength, and courage, which could be cultivated in the human personality by befriending the tree, making objects out of its body, and absorbing its characteristics by eating its flowers, leaves, barks, shoots, and roots.

In the North American Seneca tradition, trees are referred to as "the standing people" and teach humans the qualities of rootedness and giving. Trees remind us that we must maintain our connection to the body of the earth in order for us to feel rooted and able to extend our energy to others. The more seasons pass in which a tree has the opportunity to pull sustenance from the soil through its everspreading roots, the more solid and stable its trunk. Deep roots allow a tree to withstand difficult weathers and transform the minerals of the earth into the flowers, leaves, and fruits so many creatures benefit from. Akin to the trees, during winter's stillness we have the opportunity to focus our awareness down into our roots in order to encounter and anchor our foundations and to touch an inner source from which we can receive sustenance. This skill allows our giving selves to emerge fresh and renewed at springtime.

Trees have always felt like family to me. When I was a small child, wrapping my arms around a tree trunk felt like hugging my grandfather's waist. Both smelled spicy and pungent. Both seemed large, strong, and friendly. Even the hardness of the trunk which scraped my nose as I pressed the length of my young body into its thick one felt much like crawling into my Papa's lap, burrowing into his belly and hitting my face with his tie clip.

On drizzly March days I used to sit under the blue spruce in our next door neighbor's yard. The fringed hoop of its branches brought the pricking, grey-green leaf tips low to the ground, making a wide skirt I hid under. The brown earth beneath the tree was scattered with pine cones and various other treasures I examined and sometimes pocketed. More often I hid my treasures in the hollows of the tree trunk, secretly hopeful my collection would be kidnapped by a wild, unknown creature who would leave behind a trace of its identity through fur, print, or bone. I awaited also a chance to glimpse the nymphs, fairies, and elves who left gems and coins in the hidden nooks of the spruce's body. My child self was naturally and deeply fed by this fragrant being, a second mother who offered a peace I drank in urgent draughts. Under the tree, I became invisible, sheltered from rain and screened from adults as I observed the world from this secret hiding place.

I remember the long walk from the raised curb edge which delineated the neighbor's lawn to the whorl upon whorl of drooping branches that circled the trunk of the spruce. When I was in college and returned home for a visit, I was shocked to find how few strides it actually took for me to cross the lawn toward the tree. In my youth it had seemed like a knee-deep wade through a meadow. When the neighbor's house was sold, the new owners cut down the spruce to make a larger concrete porch for their quickly growing family, and I felt, for the first time in relation to the natural world, the acute pain of loss. To this day I still see the towering evergreen when I look across their lawn and the imprint of its shadowy shelter and calming silence wraps itself around me.

Many years later, when I moved to upstate New York, I felt instantly at home, for I was constantly surrounded by my tree brothers and sisters. I took my first hikes in the woods, stopping to notice the intricate motifs on treebark and the exquisite edges of leaves. In summer I tarried to enjoy the shade beneath trees; in spring I pressed my mouth against their rough skin, to taste the sap dripping out of their torsos.

Midway down the large hill into downtown was a house called Marvin Gardens, where different groups of students lived and cooked together. In the backyard of that house was the largest tree I had ever seen. It was so thick waisted that it took four people holding hands to circle it. One summer afternoon, on a day where the air was so heavy people barely spoke or moved, I was standing on the street with someone and heard a terrible scream. The wailing grew and grew, overtaking my ability to concentrate on my conversation. The cry seemed larger than human and was filled with such suffering and outrage that I began to run toward it to see if I could help.

As I came closer, I realized the cry was coming from the back of Marvin Gardens. By the time I got to the backyard, I saw the many limbs of the giant tree scattered across the ground like a hacked octopus, pieces of its body laying in a pile. All that was left as a witness to the tree's hugeness was a large stump and roots holding onto the earth like a giant claw. My heart felt as if it had been sawed in two.

I will never forget the sound of that tree crying as she was killed. It confirmed for me in the most vivid fashion that nature was alive. And the pain which tore through my body as she cried out taught me that I was and am not separate from the tree, and when she is killed, I feel her destruction.

The soul of our humanity knows that we walk upon a living, breathing organism. In the past, many traditions referred to the body of the earth as a mother, for it was clear that our wellness interpenetrated hers, as we were nurtured by many gifts emanating from her body. It was understood that if the trees were not healthy, the people could not thrive.

Without the oxygen given to us by the inhalation of the trees, we would not be able to take our next inhalation. Trees are the lungs of the earth; the health of the earth's lungs is intimately connected to the health of our lungs. The respect or carelessness we accord the trees, dependent on our view of them as either sacred or mundane, echoes our relationship to our own bodies and recreates patterns of wellness or discord in ourselves and in the environment.

In societies where this interdependency was honored, tree pruning and cutting was done in a conscious manner that persists today in unbroken tribal communities. Plants were often gathered by hand so one could physically sense, by tugging, which plant parts were ready to separate from the tree. Permission was asked of the spirit who lived in the tree to take branches from it, and an offering was often left at the base of the tree in exchange for its gift. Care was taken to preserve enough trees for the generations to come; for it was not forgotten that the continuance of our species is interwoven with the preservation of the tree family. Today, as large areas of forest are timbered for the many industrial purposes we participate in and benefit from, we are literally cutting down our possibilities for health, vitality, and the healing of our spirits offered by these "standing people."

The good news is, our kinship with the trees allows our bodies, emotions, and spirits to be deeply nourished by their healing forces. Imagine, for a moment, an old tree, rooted to the same spot for 500 years, which has been suffused by all the weathers, activities, and beings which have passed before it. When one eats from this tree one's body absorbs all that has passed through the eyes of the tree. To sit under such a tree is to rest in the presence of a knowing elder. When we view the tree this way, we begin to understand why preservation of the old trees is so important, for the ancient trees can impart to us the history, attitudes, and skills of the beings who walked peacefully on the earth. Trees carry ancestral memory much in the way the elders of our immediate families pass stories, their purpose being to connect and strengthen the links between the old and young. Trees impart their wisdom to us through the dignity of their presence; by listening deeply under the arc of their branches we can access the images and memories stored by them, remembering our roots and watering our sense of connectedness.

When we consciously use the standing people as food, medicine, and a source of ritual, we become awake to the multifaceted place these wonderful creations hold in the scheme of our lives. When we begin to relate and respond to trees as sentient beings, our concern for their well being and our commitment to their protection deepens, not out of moral responsibility but out of a love which ties our own serenity and well-being with the wellness of the tree.

Words cannot express the magic and sheer joy which has returned to my life as I have gradually learned to listen for and hear the subtle speech and wisdom of the trees and plants, called the *green nations* by the native peoples of North America. I believe that learning how to prepare teas, broths, salves, and syrups from the plants and playing beneath the trees has restored within me what I knew and cherished as a child: that nature is profoundly alive, awake, and magical, willing to reveal the many, many worlds which lie in the folds of her body to those who approach her with tenderness and respect.

Spring is nature's splendid reminder to us of life's regenerative power. Though I experienced sadness at the loss of the blue spruce because of my intimate connection to her, a young white birch tree is now growing in its stead, emanating grace and simplicity to all who wander near her slender, many-eyed trunk. I have placed birch in the month of March to honor the tasty sap of the sweet birch *(Betula lenta)* which begins to rise and flow as the new season wraps its moist and honeyed air around all that has survived the winter cold.

BIRCH *(Betula lenta, Betula alba)*

This sweet birch is known as the cherry birch, because of the similarity of its darkly gleaming outer bark, particularly of the young saplings, to that of the cherry tree. The word birch comes from the Sanskrit root *bharg^* which means "shining," for as the snow melts and sends rivers of water down the tree trunk, the birch bark indeed takes on a liquid glitter.

In the course of the spring rains, the bark becomes so wetly dark that this birch has come to be named the black birch.

The medicine of the cherry birch lies in its inner bark, which contains a rich, fragrant oil known commercially as wintergreen. The name wintergreen hints at the tree's effectiveness as a transitional herb between winter and spring. The black birch assists us in locating within our own bodies the signs of spring which have been buried under winter's white landscape. The oil aids us in shedding our protective winter layer and sprouting our green selves.

The cambium layer of the tree, directly underneath its dead, outer bark, contains this therapeutic substance which can be located by gently shaving the outer bark of the tree away with one's fingernail. The slim second layer of the tree is bright green, and one deep whiff of the bark will tell you whether you have found the birch's precious wintergreen oil, or the musty, cough suppressant medicine of cherry bark. The wintergreen oil in birch contains methyl salicylate, the plant substance from which aspirin was synthesized. This substance, both pain-relieving and anti-inflammatory, lies within the inner bark of both the twigs and branches of the silver and black birch trees. Sipping an infusion of hot black birch will ease headaches, arthritic aches, and sore muscles.

Betula lenta, the cherry birch, loves to grow near the water, giving us a signature of its gift as a tonic to the water-dependent elements of the body. Birch maintains a balance of fluids inside and outside the body's cells, the fresh sap relieving the body of excess fluid and edema. In the intestines, birch acts as a gentle laxative that simultaneously strengthens the walls of this internal pathway. Birch can be used as a tonic to the bladder and kidneys; the oil of birch, applied to the surface of the skin, relieves pain in the small of the back by the kidneys, increasing circulation in that area. Sipped as a tea, birch infusion warms and strengthens the kidneys internally.

Black birch twigs and leaves are rubefacient, quickly bringing red blood cells to the surface of an area, making a bath of birch twigs wonderful for stiff joints and general muscular achiness, particularly in the lower back region. In eastern European countries, the leaves and twigs of the birch were gathered, bound up into a broom and used in the sauna, where one's body skin was vigorously pounded with the broom-stick, bringing spring's awakening to the body in quite a literal manner! In Russia, the leaves of the white oak were similarly employed.

The blood-bringing quality of the birch makes it an excellent bath in winter for warming those areas of the body which have received too much draft or have become chilled due to contraction against the cold. Because the dried twigs and bark do not store the wintergreen oil well, an infusion of the fresh twigs and branches in oil can be made in the spring or autumn time and used in the bath during the colder months. The vitamin E in birch imparts to the infused oil an emollient, preserva-tive quality which makes birch oil regenerative to the skin. The vitamin C in the bark, accessible through sipping the infusion, increases one's re-sistance to infection. The infusion is also rich in several B vitamins.

The astringent bark of the black birch is useful in healing open sores, particularly the open, weeping wounds of poison ivy. A tea is made by boiling the leaves and twigs (nick the twigs to release some oil) and bathing the wounds in the tea. The drying quality of the twigs and the pain-re-lieving skill of the wintergreen oil ease all forms of mouth sores. A fresh twig of birch can be rubbed along the gums and used as a toothbrush.

The buds of the black and white birch, steeped for six weeks in vodka, are used for colds, rheumatic complaints, and gently relieve the kidneys of small stones. An infusion of the buds can be used for the same purpose. An infused oil of white birch is said to cure nonhereditary baldness while easing eczema and psoriasis.

The black-rimmed eyes of the white birches watch the terrain, re-minding me to serve as my own source of protection by staying alert and aware of the sounds and movements around me. In Russian folklore, a stem of birch around which a red ribbon is tied can be carried on one's person or hung in the house to ward off the evil eye. Folk were some-times tapped on their bodies with a wand of birch to dispel harmful spir-its. Birch wood was used to fashion cradles, its protective spirit keeping the fairies from coming and stealing the newborn.

In my own Russian heritage, the birch trees were deeply revered through song and story. As a child, I remember huddling next to the pink radiator in my room, wrapped in a blanket, and reading the story of

Vasalisa and Baba Yaga. The Yaga, who is the goddess of nature, was described as a great Russian hag (wise woman) who lived in the thick forest, in a house that turned round and round on chicken's legs. The simple fact of Baba's presence in the forest caused me to yearn for the wood, which in Russia, consists largely of birch trees.

In one version of the story, little Vasalisa is sent by her evil stepmother to the Yaga's house for fire. The girl ties a ribbon around an enchanted birch tree and feeds rolls to the watchdogs. In return for the gift of care, as the girl escapes from the child-hungry old woman, the birch tree refuses to poke her eyes out. The dog gives her a comb, instructing her to thrust it behind her if the Yaga should make chase. And so the witch does, flying through the air in a mortar and pestle, in hot pursuit of her warm-blooded dinner. When Vasalisa pitches the comb, it turns into a thick forest of birches which hides her from Baba Yaga's view until she is able to return home.

While eastern European folklore focuses on the protective powers of the birches, the Nordic countries consider birch (byark) the symbol of the earth mother, embodying the female, cyclical powers of growth and healing and representing the whole of the natural world. In western Europe birch is considered the Lady of the Wood, belonging to the element of water and under the dominion of the planet Venus. It is said that if one wishes to communicate with the goddess, one should sit silently in a grove of birches and listen for her whispers, which travel on the gentle gusts of the rising wind. I have had the experience of leaning my hurt back against the trunk of a slim black birch and feeling as if hands were re-patterning the energetic threads of my cells, causing the pain in my shoulder to subside.

In the Seneca tradition, the white birch (*betula alba*) is believed to teach the skill of being truthful with ourselves and learning to recognize whether others are speaking truth. The eyes in the trunk of the tree teach us to look deeply as we assess the people and situations in our lives, so that our actions come from clear vision rather than distorted perception. Creating and carrying a staff made out of the white birch is an ancient, wise way of allying one's self with these qualities. Constant physical contact with the powers embodied in the tree is nurtured and maintained by walking with the staff in hand, and alerts those who know of these mysteries to the medicine carried by the person holding the staff. Wands of birch can be fashioned and used to point the way to clear intent and fresh beginning in life as we enter the season of rebirth.

For me birch trees are enchanters of the woods. When I am amidst the white birches, I feel as though I have entered a realm of strong, united intelligence. Birch groves feel so comfortable to me that I believe them to be my second home, and the birches my second family. Often I am reluctant to end my visit with them. Their thin arms, swaying in the wind, beckon me, and seem to whisper my name through their leaves, insisting that I remain with them forever and relieve myself of the cumbersome weight of the modern world. When I soak in a hot bath seasoned with hot black birch infusion, the cares of the human world are absorbed and transformed by the refreshing, rising scent of wintergreen oil.

While it is difficult to escape the technology of this age, we can use the plants and the making of plant medicines to restore a wildness of the soul through working with our hands. Gathering the twigs of the birches, stripping the outer bark, breaking the twigs and making brews bring the rising sap of springtime into our lives. The wintergreen smell of the birch delights and awakens us while bringing us forest medicine.

∾ BLACK BIRCH INFUSION

an armful of thin black birch branches
boiled water
½ gallon jar with an airtight lid
a knife

The black birches are native to northeast America. Taking a tree identification book and searching for the trees is a worthy treasure hunt. You can also call your local park and ask if they have the trees. Over the years I have come to know the distinctive patterns of the black birch as it grows from thin sapling to majestic maturity. When you find a tree you would like to harvest, gather it in the spirit of the native peoples, leaving a gift and taking those young branches that bend easily between your fingers or would assist the health of the tree. Your hands may be drawn to some branches which snap and fall to the ground as you attempt to bend them. This is the tree's way of guiding you to help clear away her dead growth. This activity can also serve as your gift, offered in exchange for her medicine.

Once you are home with your branches, sit down at a table. Put on some music that settles you, or sing to yourself while you are working. Take a black birch in your hands and slide your knife along the outer bark to expose the cambium layer. It is nearly impossible to separate the thin, green cambium layer from the outer bark, so when you hit the ivory pith of the branch, you've gone deep enough. Nick the branches every couple of inches or so, or break up the twigs into small segments.

Every so often, cup your hands around your nose and take a deep breath. All the freshness of spring will drift through your nose to all the places within you that need this reminder. The wintergreen scent sweeps out the corners of your lungs like a broom, banishing the cobwebs of winter.

When you are finally done, place the twigs in the jar. Pour the boiled water over the twigs. Cap the jar, let it sit for eight hours, so the oil penetrates the outer bark and settles into the water. After the eight hours, you have black birch infusion. You may reheat the infusion over a low to medium flame but do not let it boil.

☙ BLACK BIRCH SPRING BATH

black birch infusion

Heat up a gallon of infusion and add to the bath water. The aromatic oils in the birch are excellent for soothing a sore lower back, for any pain in the kidney area, and for soothing aching limbs. Steep yourself in the bathtub for at least twenty minutes, and your skin will glow rosy pink with healthy blood circulation as your pains dissolve.

ᥱ᠊ BLACK BIRCH SODA

black birch infusion
sparkling water
birch sap or maple syrup for sweetening
saucepan

Place one pint of the black birch infusion into the saucepan. Place a chopstick vertically into the pan, to measure the height of the liquid. You want to simmer the liquid until it is half the amount you began with. To properly decoct an infusion, make sure the flame is quite low, so that the steam rises off of the liquid as it evaporates, but the liquid does not boil. Decocting an infusion can take anywhere from one or more hours, depending on how much liquid you start with.

After you have halved the liquid through the heating process, it will smell quite strong and have both a thicker consistency and a darker hue. Sweeten the brew with maple syrup, honey, or birch sap if you have it. Fill a glass about one third of the way with the syrup. Add sparkling water. Adjust the ratio of syrup and fizzy water to your liking.

I keep the syrup in the refrigerator (where it lasts several weeks) and add the sparkling water when I am ready to drink it.

ᥱ᠊ INFUSED BLACK BIRCH OIL

black birch branches
2 clean, dry jars, able to hold 6-10 ounces, with a good lid
(if possible, use a jar which is amber-colored)
cold-pressed olive oil
a pocket knife
a chopstick
address labels
cheesecloth

Invite a friend to help you with this, as peeling bark can be tedious even as it calms and focuses our energy. Begin to slide the pocket knife along each twig and branch of the black birch, releasing the scent of winter-green oil into the room. Solidly line the bottom of the jar with twigs, making sure to leave very little air space. When the jar is almost full, with about one-quarter inch of space left from the top, pour olive oil over the twigs to the jar's rim. Take your chopstick and press down the twigs, packing them more closely and letting the air bubbles rise to the top. Keep pressing the peeled bark until you have removed most of the bubbles. Then top off the jar again with more oil, and cover tightly.

Mark the label with the date, the name of the plant, the matrix it is steeping in, and the date six weeks from when you have begun steeping the oil. You may also include the phase of the moon in which you gathered the birch. Place the label *on the lid* of the jar.

Store the jar with a plate or tray underneath it, as the oil will seep out and down the sides as the plant releases its gases into the oil. Every couple of days for the first two weeks, open the jar, press out the air bubbles, fill the jar with extra oil if needed, and cap tightly again.

After six weeks, *decant* the oil. Take the cheesecloth and cut out a piece large enough to fit over the mouth of a clean, dry jar. As you cover the mouth of the jar, put a rubber band around it and press a bit of give into the center of the cheesecloth. Slowly pour your infused oil into this other jar, allowing the cheesecloth to catch the twigs which fall.

If you store the oil in an amber jar, it will last longer. Keep whatever jar you use in a dark, dry place. It will last in potency about a year or two. When your back aches in the wintertime, or if you strain your lower back from lifting, you can pour a generous amount of black birch oil into the bath. It will warm and ease your tired limbs as it softens and moistens your skin.

❧ Black Birch Salve

1½ ounces infused black birch oil

beeswax

vitamin E oil

a 2-ounce jar

a saucepan

Grate a teaspoon of beeswax for each ounce of oil you are using and set it aside. Heat up the black birch oil under a very low flame. If the oil begins to bubble, lift it up off the heat source. Sprinkle in the beeswax. Stir with a chopstick until it has all melted. Pour into a two ounce jar. Add three drops of vitamin E oil, which acts as a preservative. Cap the jar, and leave the salve near an open window, where it will begin to harden. Within fifteen minutes to a half hour, you will have a salve. If you like your ointments easily spreadable, a teaspoon of beeswax per ounce of oil will suffice. If you like your ointments hard, add up to two teaspoons of beeswax per ounce of oil.

Just this year I gathered birch branches in early March, when the tree was still bare. I was intending to make an oil, experimenting with using a base of grapeseed rather than olive oil, but the grapeseed oil I ordered didn't arrive. So I put the branches in several inches of water on the dining room table. Over the course of several days the buds sent out tiny papery sheaths. Within a week, these white, tissuelike membranes transformed into half-inch long, light green baby leaves. Looking at the leaves, I was reminded of the perfection of a newborn's hand. The young leaves of the birch contained all the details of a fully formed leaf: the veining, the serrated edge, in miniature form. Stroking the leaf was like touching an infant's velvet skin.

I was stunned by the power of the life force, by the fact that these cut branches had continued to sprout leafage. Though they had been cut away from the tree, it seemed that they were still connected to the mother tree, and were sprouting in my home as the still-rooted birches were unfurling their leaves in the forest I had gathered from.

BEGINNING

from winter to green, the unseen is now seen.

The uplifting cacophonous songs of the birds, the increasingly warm glow of the sun, and the sweet green smell rising like steam off the pungent, wet earth all tap on our winter shells and nudge us to break out of our winter reflections to begin the active dance of life once again. As we watch the seed sprout and the bud unfurl, something in us leaps to begin once more: to create again, love again, and contact joy as we excitedly outdistance the dark, icy winter.

Around this time of the year, one can find many stories, symbols, and rituals which enact or mark spring's homecoming. The journey of the death and resurrection of the son is honored in the Christian tradition. The Jewish Purim holiday revolves around the liberation of persecuted Jews by the wise efforts of a loyal, Jewish man and his beautiful, clever niece Esther. In pre-Christian western Europe, the Anglo-Saxons worshiped Eostre, the moon goddess of spring, at this time of the year.

Eostre's sacred animal was the moon-hare, so named by the Celts, who saw the shape of a hare in the moon's surface. This moon-hare was said to lay eggs in honor of the goddess, encouraging her to spill out her fertile energy onto the land and to all living creatures. And so the custom of decorating eggs as a symbol of the renewal of abundance and fertility was born. Following the way of the moon-hare, eggs were plunged into newly ploughed fields, buried at gravesites, and given as gifts to children, all to ensure new beginnings after winter's cycle of decay and death, and to coax the goddess of spring out of her winter sleep.

The practice of dyeing and decorating eggs was highly developed in eastern Europe. Eggs were elaborately painted with symbols of protection, strength, fertility, prosperity, and unity. These eggs, called *pysanky* and *krashanka*, were then eaten as a way of ingesting the desired quality which had saturated the egg via the magical symbols drawn upon its shell. Small, painted eggs were also worn as amulets of protection.

On the spring equinox, when the light of day and dark of night are equal in length, the Druids planted red eggs, which had been dyed to symbolize the female life force, in the fields to ensure fertility and to reap the blessings of the goddess through this offering. The red color represented the potent female womb blood which made the nurturance of newly created, unborn life possible.

To me eggs symbolize the mystery and fragility of new life. In American culture we tend to be forgetful of this vulnerability, as the eggs we buy are the product of a huge factory industry where the hens are cruelly mistreated and handled, and the eggs they lay are infertile. Before chickens were introduced into large-scale farming, the only eggs humans could eat were those laid in the nests of wild birds, which one might happen upon while burrowing pond-side in a bramble or while climbing a tree. These wild eggs were themselves decorated by nature in patterns and colors which camouflaged their presence to protect the life developing inside them.

Last summer, while visiting an organic farm, I was offered the chance to take an egg from a hen. When I went into the coop, I found an extremely alert and relaxed brown hen whose body completely draped over and hid the eggs from sight. What I thought would be a simple task became much more difficult for me. Picturing myself sliding my arm underneath the hen's warm body to pull the egg out, I connected much more clearly to what I was actually doing; taking the developing life of a new bird from its mother. Understanding this connection made me much more aware and respectful of the potency of life within the egg, and eager to ensure that my action would not disturb the balance of life.

The hen, settled atop her eggs, also reminded me that new life is warmed and nurtured in the dark, and is protected by a live, attentive creature. The quiet, still energy and body warmth of the hen seeps into the egg and allows the form within the egg to clarify. At the right time, the young chick itself breaks out of the egg, bedraggled and wet.

I love using the egg as the symbol of beginnings, because our beginnings are often ugly, tender, and fragile as a newborn bird. In March, spring itself often emerges with a battered look, wobbling between freezing rain, sudden snows, and periodic sun-filled days. The erratic March weather allows us to ruminate on what we would like to begin, as the unfoldment of the buds quickens our desire to create.

As the month passes, give some quiet time to becoming aware of what you might like to renew or begin as spring arrives. In late March, at the equinox, take a hard-boiled egg and dye it red, using either food coloring or several teaspoons of alkanet root steeped in boiling water. When the egg has cooled, write upon it what you would like to give life to, to nourish and tend throughout the spring. You may also place your intent into the egg by holding it between your palms and wishing upon it.

Find a white birch tree, the Celtic tree of beginnings, in a place where you can be relatively undisturbed. Bring a shovel, along with a red ribbon and your dyed, magical egg. Tie the red ribbon around the birch tree, taking a moment to revere the returning fertile goddess who makes all life possible. Then dig a hole at the foot of the birch and place your egg in it. Make sure the hole is deep enough so the egg will be protected. Ask the tree and the earth to help nourish what you are beginning, that it bring joy and pleasure to yourself and all beings. Bury the egg beneath the tree. Keep the location of your ritual and the act secret until summer comes, to quietly allow what you have decided to begin to gather shape and form.

As the season uncoils, you may want to go to the birch tree and sit on the spot where you buried the egg, as a hen sits atop her eggs, reminding yourself of and strengthening your intent to birth and tend that which you have asked the birch and the ground to help you begin. In the spirit of awareness which Buddhists call wakefulness, as you sit beneath the tree open your ears, nose, and eyes to the miraculous ritual of awakening unfolding before you as all beings bustle about, their preparations hastening the long-awaited arrival of the season of growth.

APRIL

❧

Growing, Nurturing, Renewing

IN THE SPRINGS of my childhood, rain ran like a comb through the maple trees and shook out the yellow clusters of their blossoms to the ground. Worms floated up from the rain-drenched soil, where they squirmed, writhed, and drowned in sidewalk puddles. The yellow maple flowers lay strewn along the ground in a delicate, lacy pattern; I tiptoed around and between them, for the sensation of my feet atop the wet blooms closely approximated the feeling of stepping on a pile of wriggling worms, which scattered on the cement in alarming profusion. Tree after tree, lime-green inchworms the exact hue of the emerging maple leaves hung suspended off silk threads that caught in my hair. I placed my fingertip beneath their tiny bodies, bidding the creatures walk across my skin, where each worm reared its back like a stretching cat and streamed forward, one inch at a time.

One of my strongest associations with the month of April is of the Seder, an elaborate dinner held on the first night of Passover, during which a tale of freedom is recited. The story, told in excerpts throughout various stages of dining and interspersed with dramatic ritual, recounts the liberation of the Jews from a long period of enslavement and their journey to safe, fertile ground. At the Passover Seder a goblet is filled with wine and placed at the center of the table, where it sits undisturbed.

This chalice is reserved for Elijah, the prophet who ascended to the spirit world in a chariot of fire.

As the youngest child it was my task, when the time came, to open the screen door to the back porch and invite Elijah in. A great believer in the spirit world, I took my job very seriously, and with a wildly beating heart opened the door. My throat was full of fear and excitement that I might feel the prophet's beating wings graze my cheek as he passed. Leaning my back against the door to hold it open, I scanned the sky for chariots and shooting stars. I stood stock still, poised for any hair-raising, skin-prickling changes in the atmosphere which might portend his entrance. After reluctantly returning to my own place at the table, I kept my eyes on the rim of his silver cup, hoping to catch a glimpse of the prophet's ghostly lips sipping the wine which had been reserved for him.

Come April, all life on earth beckons the merry spirit of spring with youthful expectancy. In March, at the equinox, the day and night experience a moment of symmetry and then brush past one another. With a graceful bow, the dark steps into the background and now light flings her doors open wide, summoning growth with her brilliance as the length of daylight begins to markedly exceed the length of dark. The warm April sun coaxes us out of our winter contraction; we slowly unfold, stretching our toes and fingers, arching our backs and shaking out our feet in response to the sun. When we open the doors of our homes and unclench our bodies, we are, in our unique ways, inviting in the spirit of spring. And of course, the more sumptuously we call to spring, the more enthusiastically she comes, infusing our beings with fiery zeal, with spiritedness and passion for life.

Early in the month the sun thaws the ground, softening the earth until the soil is loosened enough for us to work with our own hands, casting seeds and tending to their growth in communion with the energies of soil, light and water. These tasks provide priceless field experience in learning the secrets of growth and the habit of nurture. While the wild plants grow without any tending at all, our attempts to join with nature in the act of creation through the planting of seeds for food and flower instruct us in the wise habits that make certain the garden and idea, the body and soul, will grow and thrive.

GROWING

The goddess of the neolithic period was often depicted as a triple deity who manifested the qualities of the maiden, the mother/lover, and the crone. This triune deity braided the youthful, wild force of creation with the force of nurture and maturation, and the timely energy of decay, destruction and death. The image of the goddess was fashioned to remind all of the rhythms of life as beheld in nature. The mystery of life was to be found in the ever-turning and returning cycles of life, death, and rebirth.

In April it is the maiden who showers her teeming life force over the earth's creatures. In Hebrew the word for life, *chai*, is also the root of the word meaning wild she-animal *(chaiya)*, and this is how I see the spring: as a wild, untamed maiden bounding over the dark earth, her footfall touching all life with more life. Hair flying behind her, she leaves in her wake a trail of color, scent, and nourishment, her mood of wicked delight spreading across the ground like green fire. Roused by her passion, the green nations leap toward the sun, brimming with sheer joy, until everywhere we turn our heads we find life unfolding, changing shape, and blossoming, each form in nature dripping with beauty and transformed by the nurture of sun, rain, earth, and air.

The earth herself seems overtaken with desire to create for the sake of beauty and joy, unveiling at an astounding rate those creations which were conceived and protected in winter's ground-dark womb. Young, delectable leaves shoot up out of the soil, becoming chlorophyll-rich as they soak up the food of the sun's fire. Food and medicine plants carpet the ground abundantly, delighting the eyes and tastebuds with a palette of green hues and an array of distinctive earthy flavors. Daily, as light seeps into the unfurling leaves, the plants grow greener and greener with the blood of the sun. As we ingest these plants, we increase our inner fires and pulse with the blood of life, thus inspired to move through our days with the same abandon as the maiden goddess of spring.

I consider my first five years as an herbalist and gardener my maiden years, for I grew only the wild plants which traveled on the wind and chose to drop down in my garden plot. I did no tending, but trusted that whatever plants came into my garden were the ones I needed to maintain my vitality. I gathered, ate, and drank violets, mugwort, dandelion, yellow dock, and chickweed, strongly supportive wild plants for food and healing.

Allowing the plants to have their space and grow in their own way, to see what thrived and withered without human intervention was an important part of my own growth process. I needed to restore a sense of boundlessness and freedom within myself which had been lost. I had become grimy with the soot of the world, with its imposed, linear structures and limitations. Allowing the plants to do as they wanted restored my own sense of wildness. Eating wild foods arighted my body's unique rhythms and helped me develop the rooted strength necessary to stay close to the wisdom of my body's cycles. As I did this, my life began to thrive, and joy grew in my heart.

Creating room for rampant, chaotic growth to occur, allowing the wild to discover its own way, is one element of the foundation which must be laid before the habit of nurture can be cultivated further. It is during the time of letting things be that the sparks of creation are fanned into bright flames by the mothers of the wild: sunlight, moonlight, rain, wind, and soil. These join to feed the creatures of nature, helping all to grow strong roots with which to grasp rich ground. The elemental forces nourish to fruition creations which beautify the world and inspire and replenish our appetite for life.

NURTURING

In my sixth year of "gardening," the mugwort, my wild *Artemisia,* had seeded so incredibly that she began to take over the entire plot. Though the silvery backs of the mugworts were hypnotic and stirred my dream life, I could barely find the purple violet blossoms which strained to reveal themselves from beneath the thick growth of mugwort. The need for aimlessness which led me to make room for chaotic, unrestrained growth was finally fed, and new seeds began to push up from my inner ground. The wisdom of the earth nudged me to learn about another aspect of growth: nurture.

I began to look at the way the plants related to one another and to their elemental environment. I observed how certain plants died back in order to give room for others to grow, how even amongst the weeds there were hardy plants and those which needed more tending in order to thrive. This observation slowly began to guide me in the practice of creating limits to nurture abundant growth.

It is a difficult but maturing task to tend that which is growing; it is an act which asks us to cultivate a sense of watchfulness in order to deeply know the nature of the being we are assisting. The challenging task of *how* to nurture requires deep listening to an inner voice which wisely informs our decision-making. This listening necessitates courage to follow with actions that don't always instantly move us forward, but sometimes guide us to wait, cut back, pull up, and say no in order for growth and blossoming to occur. My experience with the plants has shown me that the groundwork of all growth is applying a loving hand, whether I am restraining, feeding, pulling up, or shaving back; an attitude of care causes things to live: to take root, rise up, and blossom.

This month, beside the fire of the sun lies the sometimes stormy, sometimes soft presence of rain which nourishes plant life. The patter of rainfall in late April, with its steady rhythm, penetrates me with a strong sense of security and nurturance as it fills the air with mists that hold the sweet scents of tree and ground flowers. In an air thick with moisture, we as well as the plants are transformed by the April rains. For at winter's end, we have used up our inner energies and slowed down with the freezing weather and lack of light. Though March awakens our willingness to begin, our bodies are still slow with cold, our bones creaky with winter wind.

April's wet air moistens our inner pathways, which have grown thirsty and dry from so much time indoors. To quench our thirst, the rains give rise to plants which renew our inner rivers. The wild plants that thrive in April are rich in minerals that replenish the essential waters of life: the blood and lymphatic systems. As spring takes hold, we can ally ourselves with these plants to renew the stream of life through our veins, to nourish our livers, kidneys, and reproductive organs and strengthen our digestion.

VIOLET *(Viola tricolor, Viola odorata)*

The gentle, powerful violet's wild home is in the shadowed places of the wood, where she carpets the forest floor and encircles the trees. Her dark purple flowers draw our attention downward, reminding us that we need only look to the ground beneath us to find and delight in magic, medicine, and beauty. Violet also thrives well in the garden; the rhizomes which are her horizontal roots spread out in search of shaded areas in which to unfurl her palm-size, tonguelike leaves. When the April breezes catch the underside of the violets, the leaves ripple and flutter like green hearts. The powers of violet are like the ocean: ancient, endless, and ever-creative, her healing gifts permeating into all aspects of one's being.

Some call violet, with her distinctively heart-shaped leaves, *heart's ease*, and indeed, she is a plant of compassionate heart. Violet restores the element of comfort to its primary place as a potent, transformative power in easing grief and illness. Rocking us in her watery arms, violet leaf infusion loosens tightness in the lung area, coaxing sorrow out of the chest, receiving our tears as she soothes the broken heart. Once the heart has been unburdened of pain, violet leaves and blossoms keep the heart light by strengthening our emotional expressiveness. With violet as an herbal ally, feelings flow rather than hardening or becoming trapped in the tissues of the lungs, breasts, and belly.

Violet's healing style follows the pattern of the April rain. Steady, rhythmic, and frequent, violet slowly nourishes the terrain of our bodies with vitamins and minerals. The leaves of violet have a light, bland taste and the grass-green scent characteristic of wild foods. Rich in ascorbic acid, violet leaves added to salads and soups or drunk in infusion will increase the body's resistance to infection, enhance its ability to heal wounds, and prevent headaches. Violet assists the liver in producing vitamin A, essential for strong vision, cancer protection, and good digestion.

Like the rain, violet cools and moistens the environment in which she is present, slowly dissolving hardnesses in the glandular and lymphatic channels with her flowing nature. As she slips down the digestive tract, violet nourishes and strengthens the mucus membranes, increasing bioavailability of these nutrients to the cells. Violet also acts as a gentle laxative, bringing moisture to the organs of elimination. A flower water made from violet's purple petals has been used for centuries by women for hydrating and smoothing the skin.

Violet's ability to relieve pain stems from the salicylic acid present in the leaves, which works to ease the swelling and achiness that accompany headaches, flus, and external wounds. As you munch a violet, the leaves release a sliminess that is the healing mucilage of plant. The mucilage tenderly eases discomfort as it slides past the mucus membranes lining the digestive tract, relieving the pain of intestinal and stomach ulcers. Violet infusion acts as an expectorant in the lungs, bringing up hot, yellow mucus while simultaneously moistening and cooling inflamed, dry throat tissue and shrinking swollen glands.

Wherever she applies her hand, heart's ease cools and comforts. Applied fresh to boils, burns, and hot wounds, violet brings instantaneous cooling and pain relief. This is accomplished by making a "spit poultice": chewing a mouthful of fresh violets until the mucilage is released and then applying the resulting mush directly on the affected area. Violet is a welcome balm following dental visits; a poultice can be applied to the gums, greatly reducing the pounding pain that often follows dental work. Violet infusion can be sipped as well to ease the headaches which follow the wearing off of novocaine. Fresh violet leaves soothe gum abcesses and reduce the pain and inflammation of canker sores. Frequent applications of violet cause cold sores to disappear.

Violet is under the dominion of the planet Venus, sea-born goddess of love, sexuality, and the well of feeling that matches the ocean's depth. Perhaps arising from her connection with Venus, violet has a specific affinity for strengthening and healing the sexual organs. Her effects are most notable in the breasts and reproductive system. A single cup of violet infusion greatly alleviates premenstrual breast tenderness and acts as a diuretic, reducing the swelling women feel in the breasts before we bleed. The effects of violet are enhanced when women reclaim our menstruation as a powerful time to access inner visions. Even a brief retreat from the linear demands of the world, during which we honor our cyclical, lunar rhythms and nourish solitude, deeply alters our reproductive health. Violet's tenderness matches the sensitivity of the breast tissue, where the plant diminishes the soreness of fibrocystic breasts and eases the pain of mastitis. Frequent sips of violet infusion gently dissolves benign and malignant breast cysts and tumors. Limiting one's caffeine intake is crucial for the reduction of cystic conditions.

I always suggest violet as a restorative herb to those who have suffered either a physical or emotional trauma. The shock of surgery, chemotherapy, invasive diagnostic procedures such as pap smears and biopsies and sudden loss all respond to violet's soothing energy. The hearts and wombs of women recovering from abortion are comforted by violet infusion.

For a long time the invisible but potent healing power of comfort has been pushed to the background of western medicine. The environment within which allopathic procedures take place is often sterile, cold, and frightening. Our bodies are viewed as machines comprised of parts, and the conclusions reached through technical and logistical means are trusted in place of or before intuitive wisdom. At best, we are trained to see our bodies as vehicles that sometimes break down and need fixing, and at worst, as a machine that has failed us. Often, as we begin our journeys into the world of holistic medicine, we take these familiar, deep-rooted, and unexamined attitudes with us. As soon as we feel unwell, we want options that offer instantaneous results. We rarely pause and attend to what *wisdom* our bodies may be attempting to express, through illness, that might be in the interest of our greater health, wholeness, and holiness.

Pausing to ask our bodies, in an open, heartfelt way, what they are reflecting to us through illness can bring fresh insight into our challenges and prevent us from making rash decisions about our health based on fear. This is not to say that we are wholly responsible or have somehow caused disease in our bodies. To assume total responsibility in an age of nuclear fallout and environmental toxicity is ignorant as well as merciless. But particularly when our ills are touching into the sexual and reproductive organs, great tenderness is required in our handling of matters, for the breasts and reproductive, sexual organs are the most sensitive areas of the body and can be traumatically affected by harsh methods for removing lumps, hardnesses, and cysts.

So it is encouraging to know of the less intrusive herbal option regarding growths which violet, among other herbs, provides, of *dissolving* hardnesses in the body over time as it brings immediate soothing and comfort to painful swellings. Violet steadily breaks down reproductive cysts and tumors and sends them flowing through a violet-strengthened lymphatic system to be excreted from the body. The leaves used for the infusion can then be applied warm to the breasts and belly for the same purpose.

In our culture there is a growing fear instilled into women about our breasts and their potential to nurture cancer. We learn only to touch our breasts in search of lumps and abnormalities. A weekly massage of the breasts with a salve made from violet oil can create a more loving, honoring relationship with our breasts. As we massage our breasts, we can give thanks for these organs of nurturance and pleasure and listen to the calling of our hearts. We can make room for and release the tears of old pains nestled in our breasts and wombs. We can return the gift of nurturance through the emollient, smoothing effect of the violet ointment as violet's anticancer qualities seep through the skin into the breast tissue. Violet ointment is a wonderful gift for young women with growing breasts or who are beginning their first bloods.

Violet has been noted as an ally in preventing breast cancer, and works slowly and steadily to dissolve benign and cancerous skin cysts. There have been reported incidents of violet healing internal cancers as well. The infusion or broth of violet gently eases the pain of those suffering from terminal cancers.

Violet blossoms bloom for several weeks from mid-April onward. They range in color from deep purple to white with lavender strokes on the petals and are quite delicious in salads or munched one by one. The April flower is *not* violet's reproductive flower; it is an expression of spring's riotous joy. Legend has it that violet blossoms were created by Jupiter as food for his lover Io, whom he changed into a white cow to escape his wife Juno's jealousy. Violet blossoms are rich in vitamin C and are gently laxative. The blue-purple color they impart to water, vinegar, and wine indicate their cooling effect, particularly on the throat and head, areas ruled by those colors, according to the Hindu chakra system.

Strew fresh violet and pansy blossoms in salads to restore joy and delight the senses. Use them as bookmarks and press them into books you know you'll be reading in wintertime. Decoct syrup of violet flowers to ease sore throat; infuse the blossoms in oil and drop into ringing ears, spray flower water on the back of your neck to refresh and cool the whole body. Watch your headache lift as you string violet blossoms into garlands and crown yourself the maiden of spring. To leap like the young goddess, steep a handful of blossoms in a glass of white wine. Toast to *chaiya*, and drink.

ℰ VIOLET SPRINGTIME SOUP

> *1 qt of violet leaves*
> *1 qt of curly yellow dock leaves*
> *2 cups of mallow leaves*
> *4 potatoes*
> *4 onions*
> *2 big soup pots*
> *a blender*
> *fresh garlic to taste*
> *plain, organic yogurt*

This soup needs more than one pair of hands for gathering the leaves, but the resulting brilliant green soup is highly energy enhancing.

Mallow *(Malva neglecta)* is a creeping plant with long-stemmed, round-toothed leaves. Rich in plant mucilage, mallow has expectorant qualities and adds a pleasing thickness to this soup. Yellow dock *(Rumex crispus)*, a nutritious member of the buckwheat family, has long, thin, leaves with a distinctive mid-rib. The leaves of the yellow dock curl slightly at the edges and the leaf joints are wrapped in a thin, papery sheath. Yellow dock is strengthening to the digestion and greatly increases the body's ability to absorb iron. A liver-building and digestive herb, the leaves taste tangy from the high iron and vitamin C content and wilt quickly under the effects of steam.

Boil the potatoes. When they are almost done, fill the pot with the violet and mallow leaves and add half the amount of water. Cover and steam. When they are several minutes away from tender perfection, add the yellow dock leaves.

Sauté onions and garlic separately. When the greens are tender, puree them in the blender, adding the onion mixture a bit at a time. Put the blended greens back in the first pot. When the potatoes are soft, slice and cream them in the blender with enough water so the mixture pours out like cake batter into the pot of pureed greens. Play with the consistency; you want to end up with a thick, dark green soup.

You can experiment with adding curry, lemon, or cayenne to this soup for added flavor. I prefer the soup with just a bit of pepper. I add fresh garlic at the end to strengthen my immunity, and add a dollop of yogurt in the center of each bowl of soup, in honor of my Russian-Ukranian heritage. Then I place a single violet or pansy blossom on top of the yogurt. David Winston, Cherokee herbalist, says that one's diet should consist of one-third vegetables and grains, one-third the food of one's heritage, and one-third what you love. I find this suggestion spacious and soulful in a culture which swings dramatically from self-starvation to excess.

ᥱ VIOLET LEAF SALVE

> *violet leaf oil*
> *2 ounce jar*
> *beeswax*
> *pure essential rose oil*
> *saucepan*

When you make your violet oil, following the directions for birch oil, make sure to gather fresh violets on a dry day. Leave them spread out on a flat surface for an hour or so to allow some of violet's internal moisture to dry. Then make the oil.

After six weeks, decant the oil and pour 2 ounces into a saucepan. Add a teaspoon of grated beeswax for each ounce of oil. If you are making the salve for the purpose of breast massage, a teaspoon will make a salve with a soft consistency. When the wax is dissolved, pour the warm oil into the two-ounce jar. Add a single drop of rose essential oil, or the essential oil of your choice. Roses are specific for healing the heart. Allow fifteen minutes to a half hour for the salve to thicken. Store in the medicine chest for easy access. The emollient violet salve also works well as a lip balm.

ℰ VIOLET BLOSSOM SYRUP

lots of violet blossoms
a qt jar
boiled water
honey
brandy

Gather lots of fresh violet blossoms, enlisting the aid of some children to help you pick. Prepare an infusion of the blossoms, filling your jar about halfway with fresh blossoms. Steep for two hours and strain. On the stove, using a small flame, heat the infusion until you have half the liquid you began with. Add honey to taste and one or two teaspoons of brandy as a preservative. Use by the teaspoon to heal sore throats, awaken the maiden within, open psychic vision, and heal the heart.

ℰ VIOLET MIST

spring water
an atomizer
violet blossom extract
violet leaf extract

To make the extracts, you will need one-hundred-proof vodka. Follow the directions for extract making in the October chapter. For every four ounces of water, add a dropperful of extract. Treat yourself to an atomizer worthy of violet's vanity. Spray on the forehead, the heart, and in between the breasts for immediate cooling relief. Mist the back of the neck for easing headaches. The violet fairies will chase away whatever unwanted influences are clinging nearby.

ᴇ↝ Violet Leaf Salad

2 cups of violet leaves (leave off the stems)
1 cup of dandelion leaves
½ cup violet blossoms
4 handfuls of assorted spring salad greens of your choice
3 beets
1 red onion
2 hard-boiled organic eggs

This salad is an excellent "medicine" for the immune system; it is rich in iron, and nourishes the lungs, the liver and lymphatic system.

In your assortment of spring greens, include bitter greens such as mustard, or endive to wake up your liver. I myself am partial to dandelion. Tear up the violet leaves and mix in with the other greens.

Boil the beets till tender. Cut them into chunks and allow them to cool. Bring the eggs to a boil in salted water, and continue boiling for ten minutes. Rinse them in cool water and put aside.

Arrange the salad greens in the bowl and add the now-cool beets into the middle. Sprinkle the hard-boiled eggs over the center of the beets. Arrange single circles of the red onion around the beets, taking care not to use so many onions that the greens will be overpowered. Toss a handful of blossoms over the red of the beets and the green of the leaves. After all is arranged to your sensual satisfaction, you can join the sweet taste of the beets with the earthiness of toasted sesame oil and anoint the salad with vinegar.

Saint Hildegard of Bingen, an eleventh-century German mystic, abbess, artist, and visionary, used the word *viriditas,* translated as "the greening power," to describe the vitality which lies at the root of health. Hildegard believed that the earth's body also carried *viriditas,* which emanated from the warm power of the sun. An accomplished herbalist, Hildegard wrote that human breath, warmth, blood, muscles, and bones were the physical expression of the elements of earth, water, fire, and air within the human body. The health of these channels was critical in that it was through their open pathways that the *greening* power flowed. Hildegard also noted that when human beings did not take care of the elements which charged and nourished the body of the earth, the earth often responded with eruptions, floods, and earthquakes in order to rebalance her own elemental nature, allowing the greening power to continue infusing all life on earth.

The unusual abbess delighted in the infinite creativity loosed by God upon the earth, present in myriad plants, flowers grains, fruits, vegetables, and creatures. Hildegard observed that when humans felt dried out, it was because we had lost our creative power, which she wisely saw as our umbilical cord to the divine. "Sin" occurred when we refused to renew our greening power at the wellspring of creativity. Hildegard was so devout in her commitment to the holiness of the life force that she signed her letters to other bishops "stay moist and juicy." Canonized as a saint by the church, just several hundred years later Ms. Bingen would have been fingered as a witch and burned at the stake by the same authorities who had canonized her.

In the human body, it is the endocrine system which mothers our juiciness, watering the taproot of our life force. The endocrine system, particularly our reproductive organs, release into our inner streams and organs the hormones that nourish our *viriditas*, our power to create. The liver is the organ which regulates and normalizes hormone production. The largest organ in the body, the liver weighs about four pounds. Among its over five hundred tasks, the liver filters unecessary or unhealthy chemicals out of the blood. In city environments in particular, the liver works tirelessly to transform and dispose of the rather high levels of chemical contamination present in the air. The liver also adds many necessary nutrients, hormones, minerals, and chemicals into the bloodstream which are vital for the overall functioning of the body. A versed teacher in the art of nurture, the liver carries the wisdom of putting things in their proper place and of knowing when to limit or encourage growth.

Many nonwestern systems of healing view the liver as the "house of the soul," or the "seat of life." When functioning optimally, this organ keeps emotions moving, replenishes energy, and gives access to the greening power Hildegard speaks of, which I see as the potent, fertile power of the life force. Eating one's "bitters," the strong-tasting greens which encourage digestion and nourish the liver, prevents emotional bitterness, give one the ability to digest some of life's more difficult trials, and replaces depression with soul-building expression. The spring sun pulls out of the earth one of the most common, nutritive, and beautiful, bitter plants of the wild: the common dandelion.

DANDELION   *(taraxacum officinale)*

A supportive plant in the deepest sense, dandelion's relationship to the human body is one of loyalty, sustaining us in times of health and restoring us in difficult periods. The gifts of dandelion reach down into the sturdy brown fingers of its roots, permeate the rosette of its toothy leaves, and radiate out its thousand-petaled yellow flower head. Dandelion leaves are highly nutritive, the roots alterative, reversing a wide variety of ills from liver damage to depression. Through dandelion's effects on the liver, the leaf and root tone the stomach, gall bladder, pancreas, and the entire digestive tract. The flowers and stems are diuretic, nutritious, pain-relieving, and skin-healing.

It is no accident that dandelion grows so abundantly in places which are heavily populated. Though we imagine that the cures for our ills are complicated, exotic, and expensive, often the plants which are meant to be our constant companions love to settle at our feet. These plants are extremely beneficial to our vitality and resiliency. In the case of dandelion, nature has placed in our midst an exceptionally healing food and medicine plant. I find it both comical and tragic when I see humans pouring chemicals onto our lawns in order to exterminate this plant, so key to our *viriditas* and such a sun-filled feast for the eyes. A medicine for the ground as well, dandelion creates drainage pathways in compacted dirt, aerates the soil, attracts earthworms, and remineralizes earth depleted by pesticides and herbicides. As environmental pollution taxes the body's filtering systems, dandelion strengthens the liver and kidneys to transform and filter the stressful by-products of technology-laden city life.

The name *dandelion* derives from the French *dents-de-lion*, referring to this weed's deeply serrated leaves which resemble lion's teeth. Dandelions are also affectionately called swine's snout, and priest's crown, for when the petals close to allow the seeds in the ovaries to ripen, the shape of the flower head resembles a pig's snout, and when the head is denuded of it's many floating seeds, its bald appearance calls to mind the shorn scalps of medieval priests.

The bitterness one tastes upon biting into dandelion leaves gives way to sweetness as the plant's minerals begin to blend with the mouth's digestive juices. The leaves of dandelion are extraordinarily nutritive, containing rich amounts of iron, calcium, vitamin C expressed as ascorbic acid, and the vitamin B complex. For those with less adventurous tastebuds, soaking the steamed leaves in vinegar, honey, and olive oil overnight or drizzling vinegar over the leaves diminishes dandelion's initial bitter taste. A six-week vinegar infusion of dandelion will impart to the matrix the full magnitude of its vitamin and mineral power. Dandelion also provides us with vitamin A, trace minerals, and choline, essential for liver functioning. Given this impressive list of nutrients, its hard to believe someone would attempt to annihilate a plant of such character!

Beginning one's foray into the land of wild foods by eating three wild dandelion leaves a day will bring about a marked increase in vitality by the end of even one month. Eat the fresh leaves or sip a teaspoon of dandelion vinegar with each meal to reverse anemia, enrich breast milk, and reduce premenstrual sugar cravings. Dandelion is a fitting ally for women in need of high levels of absorbable calcium during the menopausal years, and vital in the prevention of osteoporosis. The calcium present in dandelion leaves and imparted to the vinegar has a calming effect on the body, smoothing out nerves as we move through stressful periods.

The leaves and spring roots, rich in taraxacin, increase the presence of hydrochloric acid in the stomach, heightening the flow of gastric juices and assuring swift, easy digestion of even rich foods. Swiss herbalist Maria Treben recommends fresh stems of dandelion for almost miraculous relief of chronic liver inflammation, glandular swellings, gout, and rheumatism. A two-week, daily course of ten fresh stems allays fatigue, removes gallstones, and increases one's energy level. I have experienced renewed digestion as well as restored visual acuity through a month-long course of the stems.

Daily inclusion of dandelion greens into the diet over a period of three months can completely clear night blindness and restore peripheral vision. This may perhaps be due to the rich vitamin A content present in the leaves, which improves eyesight by strengthening the liver.

Dandelion leaves, blossoms, and roots are tonic to women. Through dandelion's support of the liver, hormones are released in their proper rhythm, regulating the endocrine system. Dandelion root is helpful as maidens make their menstrual transition to womanhood. During this period, hormonal fluctuations often express themselves through skin eruptions; here dandelion balances the hormones, lessening the occurrence of adolescent acne. Ritual is also helpful for girls making this leap; to have an intimate group of women welcome and support one's beauty and power greatly strengthens a young woman's sense of her own sacred nature and builds self-respect. A regular course of leaf and root infusion can bring back a woman's menstrual cycle, even if it has disappeared completely for many years as a result of anorexia, heavy exercise, or rigorous ballet training.

Dandelion leaves and flowers, soaked in boiled water and applied to the breasts, ease premenstrual tenderness and soften fibrous and thickened breast tissue. Dandelion blossom ointment can be massaged regularly into the breasts for the same purpose. Dandelion blossom oil draws out emotions which have been stored in the muscles. Drinking the juice of fresh dandelion leaves is a more dramatic technique for working with fibrocystic breasts. Dandelion encourages expulsion of the placenta during childbirth, and imparts rich nutrition to breast milk.

Dandelion flowers are also highly nutritious, calmative, and strengthening to the solar plexus. Each petal of the dandelion's head is actually a whole flower, containing all the reproductive parts. Each head accommodates many tiny yellow flowers, which join to form the exquisite, sunfilled bright blossom. Dandelion flowers steeped in boiled water and applied to the face hydrate the skin, dissolve freckles, tighten pores and ease adolescent acne. The blossoms in tea relieve headaches, stomach aches, and menstrual cramps, and a breakfast of dandelion blossom pancakes dissipates lethargy and restores physical power. The blossoms, steeped in white wine for an hour or two, nourish digestion and bring deep, rejuvenating sleep.

In the fall, the bitter taste of the spring-dug roots and leaves turns into a mild sweetness as dandelion sends its starches, sugars, vitamins, and minerals down into the root for storage. The fall-dug dandelion root possesses the most mature expression of the plant's many gifts. Inulin, dandelion's starchy sugar, makes up one-quarter of the root's weight in the fall, offering us strong medicine for the stomach, intestines, and liver. The inulin helps balance the body's blood-sugar level, easing hypoglycemia and tapering the mood swings which often accompany sugar imbalance.

The diuretic and deobstruent qualities of dandelion root tone the kidney's filtering abilities, dissolve kidney stones, and strengthen kidneys weakened by diabetes. While allopathic diuretics tend to deprive the body of potassium, disturbing the electrolyte balance, dandelion acts in a more balanced way, imparting a generous level of potassium to the bloodstream. Dandelion root is also effective in easing chronic edema, and strengthens the kidneys and liver which have been stressed by over-consumption of coffee. Our culture's extreme abuse of the coffee plant has taken its toll on the adrenal glands, affecting our stress level and deeply exhausting the body's filtering systems. Sipping a tea of roasted dandelion root can satisfy the body's craving for bitterness without damaging the kidneys and liver.

Taken over a six-to-nine-month period, dandelion root tincture or infusion rejuvenates damaged liver tissue, making it a prime choice in healing those suffering from drug or alcohol withdrawal. Dandelion is a wise choice for those recovering from chemotherapy, radiation, hepatitis, or jaundice. The root dissipates swelling of the bile duct, and dissolves cholesterol-based gall stones. Dandelion eases indigestion, alleviates constipation, and restores strong elimination through the mineral richness of its roots. Dandelion root tincture also eases headaches which stem from overconsumption of rich foods. For situations in which the body has suffered tremendous loss of vitality, resulting in an inability for the digestive tract to assimilate and absorb nutrients, a course of dandelion and burdock root *(Arctium lappa)* steadily brings back inner strength.

In traditional Chinese medicine, the liver and gall bladder house the emotion of anger. Whether one experiences flashes of rage or cannot seem to summon anger in appropriate situations, dandelion is a wonderful ally for assisting anger to flow through us in a balanced manner, preventing anger and resentment from hardening within or turning into paralyzing sadness. Sometimes, as consistent use of dandelion nudges up old rage, one can feel overwhelmed by the power of this emotion. It is advisable to have a source of support such as a therapist or spiritual counselor who can offer guidance in transforming rather than simply discharging anger.

All parts of dandelion lift the veil of depression. For those who are spirit weary, this wild carrier of spring's maiden energy searches for and feeds the flame of strength within us, giving us the fortitude to pull ourselves up from the pit of deep despair which sometimes immobilizes us. Dandelion restores the threads of our desire to live and thrive, to create and procreate. Sluggishness slowly gives way to motivation, bitterness dissolves, and joy once again becomes possible.

For this purpose dandelion focuses its sun-drenched power on the area of the solar plexus, at the base of the ribs. The solar plexus is the home of the stomach, liver, and pancreas, organs all beneficially strengthened by consistent use of dandelion. Emotionally, an energized solar plexus gives us the power to speak our truths, manifest our visions, and respond to injustice. Swallowed rage, fear, and anxiety can tighten this area, in which case dandelion slowly works to restore the warmth and radiance of the shining sun to the solar plexus region.

Dandelion's bright yellow blossoms are very sensitive to light and weather conditions, closing up their heads in the face of impending darkness and storms. Dandelion is a wonderful ally for those with a similar emotional constitution, whose hearts open fully and joyously when warmth and light are beamed upon them, but who wither and shut down quickly when more turbulent emotions are expressed in their presence.

Dandelion is under the dominion of the planet Jupiter, which encourages expansiveness. My favorite way to experience this energy is to find and wander through a field of dandelion blossoms, pick a handful, and lie outstretched on the earth, my body open to the sun. I place two flowers over my eyes and allow my mind to wander, soothed by the drone of the bees collecting pollen. Dandelion reminds me to call on the power of light, warmth, and sweet scents to refresh the flower that lives within me.

୧ DANDELION PANCAKES (SERVES 4)

2 cups of whole wheat flower
4 tsp baking soda
pinch salt
2 eggs
1 cup water
4 tbs olive oil
2 cups dandelion flowers

Mix the dry ingredients together. Beat the egg in, then add liquid and oil. Heat the oil and stir in the flowers. Spoon batter into a hot pan and cook like pancakes. Serve with maple syrup, yogurt, or jam.

These will make you, all at once, strong thighed, sure-footed, able to stand your ground, putting your hands on a thrust-out hip to attract attention. You'll see situations clearly, and be able to stand what you see on solid legs.

The pancakes will also gently but firmly awaken your digestion.

୧ DANDELION POTATO SALAD

5 cloves garlic, minced
5 potatoes
2 diced onions
apple cider vinegar
4 cups chopped dandelion leaves and stems
toasted sunflower seeds
1 cup frozen peas

Boil the potatoes. When they are almost tender, sauté the diced onions and garlic in olive oil. When the onions are transluscent, add in the chopped dandelion leaves and stir until all the leaves are coated. Add a bit of water and cover the pot, steaming the leaves until tender.

Pull the skins off the potatoes and cube them. Fold in dandelion greens, sunflower seeds, and toss in apple cider vinegar to taste. I like to slowly add the vinegar, to make sure I don't put in too much. You may also use the herbal vinegar of your choice here. Add the peas just before serving. You may serve this at room temperature.

℮ DANDELION BLOSSOM OIL

cold-pressed olive oil
grapeseed oil
dandelion blossoms
a jar to hold what you've gathered

Gather the blossoms at noon, when the flowers carry the height of the sun's power and are sure to be dry. Make sure you fill the jar completely with blossoms. In a separate measuring cup, mix grapeseed and olive oil together, enough to fill your jar. Pour over the flowers. Use your chopstick to press out all the air bubbles. Cap and label. Keep in a dry, dark area, not too warm, as the dandelion blossoms are especially susceptible to spoiling. As the gases from the blossoms release, the oil tends to leak heavily. Open the jar every couple of days for the first two weeks, press out the air bubbles, refill the oil to the top, and cap tightly.

After six weeks, decant your oil, following the directions for other infused oils. To make salve, use a teaspoon or so of beeswax for every ounce of oil you melt.

RENEWING

Our culture operates in a linear fashion, imploring us to ignore the cyclical nature of life. We are encouraged to work at unfulfilling jobs for the sake of security and to spend our leisure time recovering from or numbing ourselves to the stress created by performing too much work without soul. As we encounter the vital spirit of spring we may find ourselves face to face with a weariness that stems from emotional barrenness rather than from winter's biting cold. It is crucial to listen to the voice of our exhaustion, and to find simple ways to replenish ourselves. As the April weather wavers between draft and warmth, we can spend some conscious time renewing our spirits, filling ourselves with the potent, fertile energy of the earth.

Climbing and laying in trees is the most magnificent, simple, and delightful secret to renewing one's energy. The very structure of trees enables them to soak up and store the powerful vitality of the sky and the earth. The power of trees to care for us was known amongst earth-based cultures in Europe and the Americas, where it was common for children to have trees planted for them at birth, or to have a tree designated as their tree. The umbilical cord from a child's birth as well as the afterbirth was often buried beneath this tree. The tree then became the guardian of that person for life. The person would cultivate a lifelong relationship with the tree similar to one's connection with a grandparent. The tree provided its body, presence, and silent speech for comfort, security, and counsel.

Sometime in the month of April, find a large tree, one you can lean your back against, climb, or lay upon. As you are doing errands, listen inwardly for any pull toward a particular direction which might lead you to the tree. Once you find it, stand away from the tree and take it in with your eyes, much the way you would a beautiful vista. You will notice that in the very stance of the tree lies a particular quality, such as solidness, strength, lightness, or grace. When you are away from the tree, practice calling the tree to mind while you are doing another activity which does not require your full attention. See if you can surround or call into yourself the feeling of the tree.

Then choose a day when you can take ample time to visit the tree. If you are a mother with children, you may have to do a bit of planning ahead. If it is possible, check a moon calendar to see when the moon is waxing, that is, growing to fullness, and take your day during the expansive part of the moon cycle.

Dress comfortably on your day off, wearing shoes you can take off easily. Take a flask of water with you and walk to the site of the tree. Pour the water in a circle around the tree, as a way of honoring the many gifts trees bring us. Then, if you can, climb the tree to a place where you can lean your spine against its trunk and rest the soles of your feet upon it. It you cannot climb, I find the best way to receive the power of the tree is to lay on my back with the soles of my feet against the trunk, or to sit upright, my spine supported by the tree's spine. As you lay in the tree, allow your body to relax completely, consciously releasing any tensions and winter tiredness into the trunk. You may feel a heaviness move through you as you do this, followed by a sensation of emptiness.

Eventually you will begin to feel your body being filled, becoming more solid, like the trunk of the tree. Mentally open the pores of your skin to the tree, allowing yourself to soak up and store its vibrant energy. If you are laying on your back on a thick branch, you may want to turn onto your belly and repeat the exercise.

As you commune with the tree, listen to the wind moving through its young leaves and branches. You may hear a whisper, or a word, meant for you. You may feel yourself blending with the tree, becoming part of her body. When you feel revitalized, slide carefully out of the tree, and bid it farewell. I usually bow in thanks.

Eating and making various herbal potions with dandelion and violet during the month of April is sure to fan your playfulness, if not your zest for growth and life. Remember, while working with the recipes follow your experimental nature, enjoying your mistakes. Almost every detail of information I offer about making herbal preparations has come through mistakes I have made and an attitude of inventive lunacy. My first pull toward herbs came from a book I read as a child, where the main character stumbled into a room of jars full of different colored powders which he then used, turning himself into various creatures and propelling himself through a multitude of historical periods. I still have the same attitude while working with salves, tinctures, and herbal food preparations. I believe the maiden of spring charges around in search of similar mischief, leaving trails of beauty behind her.

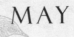

MAY

Marrying, Opening

IT IS THE beginning of May, and as I walk down Fifth Avenue beside Central Park, I see that I have an entire hour of leisure before my next appointment. Grateful for my good fortune, I enter the park's wide threshold at Ninetieth Street, passing between two stone walls. I nod to the elm tree, whose great trunk swells with watermelon-sized burls and whose roots erupt out of the cement, grasping the earth with her woody claws. The elm stands firm on her thick body, slightly set back off the park's internal, paved road, as if she were guardian of this eastern entrance to the sacred ground of Central Park.

I stop to inspect the elm's trunk, my eyes drawn to a long, blackened gash in its side. Several years ago, a group of women herbalists I know sat with this tree, for it was not well. Some strange substance other than sap had been oozing out of the great wound in its flank, weakening the tree's life force. The sickness of a mature elm was especially disturbing as many great old elms have been succumbing to Dutch elm disease, and tree cutters have had to take the lives of some large, mature elms in order to prevent contagion. For those who recognize and care about the handsome, lithe-limbed elms, the life of each remaining tree has grown precious.

The women spent some time in a circle beneath the elm, humming softly to weave a web of healing, asking the tree questions, and quietly waiting for a response to grow out of their silent listening. The women mutually discovered that indeed, the tree was the gatekeeper to this side of the park, responsible for fending off destructive energies by using its own body as a shield; the position of the tree made it highly susceptible to the toxic exhaust of passing vehicles, and the fumes were slowly depleting the tree's immunity.

The herbalists decided to apply a healing salve to the trunk of the tree. They patiently spread an herbal balm over the entire gash, and wordlessly vowed to visit the tree each time they were in the neighborhood. Now, as I touch the trunk, I see the darkened area of the old wound and that it has healed, leaving a scar that adds to the unique, elderly beauty of the tree. I give silent thanks, my brow against the elm's ample trunk, to my sisters for caring, and to the tree for its unceasing guardianship, and then I step away.

Veering off to the right, I step onto the horse path, my shoes sinking into the soft skin of the earth with each footfall. As I gaze ahead, the trees on each side of the path arch their arms as if reaching toward one another. The pink petals of the cherry blossoms and the white blossoms of the apple swirl in the air, wrapping me in a mist of flower light as the wind blows through the trees and the petals confetti the ground. The scent of the air is so sweet that my whole body is filled with the desire to open. My chest expands and my breath deepens in an effort to reel these smells in, as if my body could store this moment's pleasure in the hollows of my lungs, as if I could become the perfume of these flowers.

As I stroll languidly down the path, my feet take me to a tree with white blossoms arranged in a cluster of five-petaled flowers, some closed tight like pearls, others open and revealing pink-tinged anthers. One deep inhalation of these earthy, spiced flowers and I know I am in the presence of the great hawthorn, tree of the May. Stepping back, I take a moment to admire the tree's spiked, inch-long thorns and jagged, pointed leaves. Retreating yet a few steps more brings the tree's trunk into view, its girth the width of a mature python, the bend of its limbs curved upward and outward like a dancing serpent.

As I look into the flower clusters, I see the round, red berries which will come of these blossoms when the bees and the weather do their work; I look forward to the fine, heart-strengthening brandy I will make of its leaves, blossoms, and berries. But for today, it is enough to walk under the trees, and to rest in the green lap of the earth. I will have other days this month when I can return with my basket and gather.

Later in the week, an odd phenomenon occurs. The spring rains which suffuse the flowers and fill the air with honey-sweet scent dwindle and cease; the weather dramatically changes course and we are given several days of almost hundred degree weather. My body is confused and begins to crave ice cream, oceans, and fireflies. It is so hot I want to flee indoors, but wherever I go I am walking into "air-conditioned" spaces, cold as meat freezers, and when I enter the outdoors, the cement reflects a temperature more suited to baking cookies than to engendering life.

As the month passes, the days are hot. Flowers open before their usual time, and I hear some people grumbling about having no spring. Others seem to welcome the premature summer, as if the cold of winter was an annoying occurrence they would rather do without. My own body freezes and thaws several times daily, and the stress brought about by the swinging temperature weakens my immunity. My nerves feel like cracked eggshells. Slowly, the weather begins to drop into the eighties, and finally back to more springlike tones. By the time I have energy enough to return to the hawthorns, their petals are dried, burned at the edges, and I am unsure if the bees have done their work.

I am disturbed. I am more than disturbed. I feel despair. I am writing about my trust in the rhythms of nature, how they guide, sustain, and nourish us, and these rhythms are askew. To ignore mentioning this increasing arrythmia on the part of the earth would be an act of denial, and it is our denial, on so many levels, which has brought us to create technologies which have caused the unbalancing of the earth's cyclical fluctuations. For days I cannot write. It is as if an enormous stone is in my path, so huge that I cannot see around it, and I cannot bypass it. What can I do? I ask myself. I must sit with the stone, my heart answers, as I would sit with a plant before gathering, if I desire to penetrate, dissolve, or move past it and write again.

I put down the writing, though it hovers near as the ghost of a newly dead relative. In my being, there is a tumult which mirrors the extreme weather. Inside I feel like a field whose trees have been uprooted and toppled by the winds of a great hurricane. In the silence of this field, barren of seed, I sit with overwhelming fear that it is too late, that these rhythms, the trusty cycles which are the food of our souls, will no longer sing us their song. I am filled with a desire to abandon the earth out of a sense of powerlessness and anger. And in the clenched fist of my anger I find fear. Fear that, as a consequence of our destructive actions and our neglect, my Mother is taking her beauty away, this beauty which has so nourished, fed and filled me and which I have so loved and celebrated.

And as I continue to sit with the great, gray stone of my despair, I hear a voice from within the boulder. Not human, the voice is deep, sonorous, and utters simply: "I will not die now. And I will not leave you, though I will belch, groan, writhe, shiver, and grow feverish as I ail to renew myself." And the voice says, "Look to the hawthorn. Through the hawthorn you will see the path; you will remember the rhythm. Through the hawthorn you will find the way."

And so I gather myself up from the foot of this stone. Where I live, there are many oak, sycamore, and hawthorn trees, protected from the fumes of vehicles by tall buildings. And as my eyes search and find the first hawthorn tree, I see another. And another. And in the distance, I recognize the hawthorns by the dance of their snakelike trunks; from afar their leaves seemed to be shrouded in white. In white? Why, they must be flowering hawthorns, within walking distance of my own home!

I exhale with relief. Not all the tree blossoms have been burned by the heat. Here are several trees, one after another, arranged as if they were picnicking cousins, all just beginning to flower, in the middle of May. Bring your basket down, they say, and sit. Lay your head against our trunks, cock your ear and listen. We will tell you the story so that you may remember, that you may know what is needed and guide others in how to restore joy, come into the natural cycle, and ensure return.

I sit beneath a tree, my back against her trunk. The mid-May wind lifts up the underside of its leafing branches and there is rustling all around me. The wind exhales, pauses and inhales, each out-breath jostling the tree's limbs. I rest my spine against the tree, finding that curve in the tree's trunk, tender as the arch of a woman's foot, into which my head fits perfectly. I close my eyes, my basket beside me, listening to the breath of the wind and the foreign tongue of the trees. My ribs widen and thin with the cadence of my own breath. Images begin to spin and thicken, gathering in my mind like the clouds of a summer storm. As I look up, through my closed lids, into the flowering boughs of the hawthorn, they join themselves in my mind into a wreath. And as I see the boughs bound to form a circlet, I suddenly remember another union, a deep entwining which was once celebrated in May, known by those who practice heathen ways as the Sacred Marriage.

MARRYING

Many, many years ago, when the calendar followed the wax and wane of the moon and women marked time according to the monthly shedding of their shiny, garnet mantles of uterine blood, the first of May was a day of celebration, a day of ritual known as Beltane. Beltane was named after a Druid sun god called Belenos, who, awakened by the flowering, spring scent which wafted through the air behind the earth goddess's every movement, descended from the sky and asked for her hand. Warmed by the radiant heat of his extended palm, stirred by the light of his eyes, she took his fingers in her own. These two offered themselves to one another in marriage, vowing to endure all weathers together, and to return eternally, year after year, to renew their commitment to fertility. The seeds sown of their lovemaking gave birth to the shadowy forms of fruits which grew plump and full on the sky food of sun and rain, and ripened to fit the palms of human hands as summer deepened into fall.

But this holiday could not occur without a similar vow on the part of humans, a vow sung and danced around trees and sealed through human mating upon the freshly plowed and seeded fields. The two-leggeds made a game of running through the forest in search of the perfect tree, which from previous hunts they knew would be found lying heart to heart with the ground, and whose powerful, solid form resembled the phallus of the virile male. When the tree was chosen, it was carried out of the woods, laid upon the ground, and decorated with white and red ribbons. These ribbons symbolized the streaming forces of life and death which danced together to create new life.

The humans then knelt upon the ground and dug gently into the soil with their hands, slowly carving a deep hole to represent the holy womb of the earth mother. Finally, the people lowered the tree into the open place they had fashioned out of the earth's substance, and crowned the top of the now upright tree with a wreath of hawthorn blossoms, leaves, and thorns. Gathering up the ribbons, young and old danced round and round the tree, singing of the marriage of earth and sky, of the ever re-turning cycle of regeneration, and of the glorious flowers which would miraculously swell into fruit come autumn's harvest.

It was believed that these dances energized the soil and awakened the earth's desire to create, and so people danced deep into the night, their stomping feet arousing yet another land—the inner fields of their own desires. Slowly, couples took hands and disappeared into the far fields and thickets, the juices of their own lovemaking fertilizing the soil in the manner of the god and goddess.

In this way, humans married themselves to the earth, promising to bear with her through her cycles of life, death, and rebirth. The humans who honored this vow, bending close to the earth that they might learn the mysteries of her rhythms and seasonal cycles, grew tough-skinned and plump-fleshed like fruits. They were deeply fed and imprinted with the wild beauty which comes from refusing to abandon, from *staying with* a relationship in all its weathers. The awareness of change cultivated among the people by the seasonal honoring of the earth's rhythms of growth, decay, and regeneration built an enduring love and respect for nature. The health of the earth and all that sprouted from her body was carefully guarded and tended, as one would care for a family member.

A gust of wind ruffles the tree and nudges me gently back to present time. I muse on what I have seen in my inner visions. I think about the sacred marriage, and what it means in relation to the despair I have been feeling. I am moved by the forbearance of the people who, like the tree chosen to become the maypole, lived side by side with the earth. If I see the earth as a lover, I see that this quality of steadiness in relation to the earth is greatly needed as she swings between extremes on the path toward restoring her own rhythm.

We can assist the earth by trusting her ability and manner of finding balance. We can support the earth by staying solid in our own physical rhythms, aligning our cycles, as much as we can, with those of the earth, moon, and sun. We can honor and experience the inward, visionary power of the female menstrual time. We can listen and heed what makes our bodies flush with vitality and turn from that which diminishes our spirits. As we learn to carve out a time of rest within ourselves, we will not demand of the earth that she give constantly, pouring chemicals into her bloodstream which ultimately weaken the matrix supporting all life. If we join with others in community to celebrate the precious gifts of fertility and sexuality, we publicly avow our *joyful* responsibility toward this magical, wild being whose body we tread upon.

We can use the plants of May to lighten and strengthen our hearts, to give us the mature human powers of flexibility and fortitude to bear with the earth as she finds her way back to elemental clarity. The plants I have chosen for May carry thorns and stingers as well as fragrant flowers, tasty leaves, and edible berries, mirroring the connection of a maiden sensibility of abundant beauty and gaiety in our relationship with the earth to a growing, mature union akin to that of the sky god and earth goddess. This marriage with the earth builds within us a strong character which can tend to the more thorny, wounded face of the earth and ultimately enriches the ground of our beings, allowing a thick-rooted, enduring love relationship with nature to form.

STINGING NETTLE *(Urtica dioica)*

In the herbal tradition in which I apprenticed, great value was given to the notion of using *simples,* working with a single plant, over a long period of time. The shortest period for studying a medicine plant in depth was a year and a day. The plant usually selected the herbalist, calling to us in dreams or appearing mysteriously in our gardens and window boxes, in the planters we arranged on fire escapes. Sometimes these plants sprouted up right outside our doorsteps, where we stumbled over them on our way out.

During this year, we were encouraged to spend as much time as possible with our chosen plant, visiting it in all seasons until we could identify it as distinctly by its winter skeleton as well as spot it from a distance out of the endless maze of spring green. Young and mature leaves, flowers, root, and seed were examined, tasted, and used in a variety of ways to experience their particular effects. We played games to hone our skills, blindfolding ourselves as we tasted various preparations made from the plant, sensitizing our taste buds and noses to the various flavors of the green allies. In this way I was guided to practice becoming deeply aware of my body as well as the effects of the herbs, both on a physical level and also a spirit level. The medicine of the plants was not just for our physical well being, but often gave gifts of emotional strength which made possible the letting go of long-held anxiety and trauma in the body.

We were also encouraged to be inventive and playful in our experiments, brewing concoctions and preparations that spontaneously occurred to us, and sharing them with one another, confirming the effects of our elixirs on other willing subjects. In this way, we were building a body of knowledge which added late–twentieth century folklore to the already wisdom-laden "old wive's tales" spun in older herbals, that passed down methods of healing from grandmother to daughter to granddaughter, and in some cases, from grandfather to child and grandchild. Honing in on one plant, I found that a single plant's powers stretched in many directions and took many joyful years to discover through personal experience.

Allowing the wisdom and great gifts of a single herbal ally to unfold over a period of years can weave a link between humans and the plant world that heals the grief of our separation from nature. When seen simply as objects for our use, there is little that distinguishes an herbal cure from an allopathic one. When related to as subjects with their own dreams, desires, strengths, and gifts which we then ingest, an entire dimension is added to our healing and the myth of plants as beings of inferior intelligence is dispelled.

Quite to the contrary, because the plants retain their umbilical cord to the earth, they carry not only the earth's mineral richness and vitality, but the memories of ancient mysteries lodged within the body of the earth. When we approach the green nations with the awe and wonder of a child, and the respect of an elder, the plants slowly reveal these secrets to us. I have come to see that when I cultivate a personal relationship with a plant, it allows me to use it for working with a variety of challenges, including those outside its known scope. A single plant or tree can provide the necessary strength to its human friend over a lifetime.

Stinging nettle was my first ally. When I hear the plant's name, my heart is filled with the love and gratitude one feels for the person who has been the source of deepest support in one's life. In one of the first plant classes I ever took, this plant was served as a tea. I remember sitting on the back porch where the class was being held, listening to the rustle of the quaking aspen leaves as I sipped tea from a spotted, earthenware mug. The tea slid down my throat like silk, and my lungs opened to deeply inhale the rising steam. The smoothness of this green liquid filled my whole abdomen with a warm strength that made me let out an involuntary *mmmmmmm*. As I looked around me, the colors and shapes of the leaves grew vivid and the light danced gold upon them; my vision was heightened by this plant's green magic.

During the class, I learned that nettle was particularly supportive of the bladder and urinary tract and I instinctively knew that this plant could help me. From the time I had been a child, I had suffered from a weak bladder and kidneys. Over the course of eighteen years, I experienced the discomfort doctors associated with urinary tract infections: burning sensations, scanty urine, a need to use the bathroom but no flow, and a dull ache in my lower back on the right side. I rarely slept through the night and antibiotics seemed to do nothing to change the situation. I had gotten to the point where I was simply resigned to never sleeping well, and to experiencing urinary tract irritation if I drank any coffee or fruit juice.

I decided to try stinging nettle infusion. Within a single week, I was sleeping through the night. Within one month, all of my symptoms had disappeared. Within six months, I began to actually feel that my bladder muscle was strong. I have never experienced a urinary tract or bladder infection again. For the first week of using nettle, I added 2 dropperfuls of echinacea extract to each cup of infusion to take care of any infection that may have been present. Beyond alleviating the discomfort in my bladder, the nettles began to positively affect my general health. My head hair began to look healthy and thick, and my general sense of well being and energy grew. My resistance to illness increased, my skin began to glow, and the pain in my right kidney disappeared.

After drinking stinging nettle infusion for a year, I was impatient to meet the plant. I was out in Delaware, and as we whizzed along the road I spotted a field of nettles by its dark-green color. We stopped the car. I was so excited I waded straight into the patch, forgetting about the stingers which cover the leaves and stalks. I howled and began running out of the thicket. The stingers on the nettles raised itchy blisters on my punctured skin. Needless to say, my fall into the nettle patch was unforgettable; I now always approach *slowly* (and with a pair of gloves).

The word *nettle* derives from the Anglo-Saxon word for needle, referring to the pin-pricking hairs that cover the leaves and stalks. A Native American tale tells that nettles were created with stingers to prevent overharvesting of the plant; they were seen as so beneficial, that human beings would quickly have harvested all the nettles on earth if the stingers were not there to keep us in check. The presence of the stingers has taught me to touch the plant with care or I will quickly be reminded of how nettle likes to be handled. Nettle is a fitting ally for those who tend to be swayed easily by others, suffer from being "nice" all the time, or need to develop a more barbed tongue to protect themselves. In the Wessex dialect of the tenth century, nettle was called *wergulu* and was listed as one of the nine sacred herbs used in casting spells of protection and to reverse evil charms.

Gathering nettle has helped me practice the skill of attentiveness. If I give my full attention to each stalk I harvest, I can sometimes pick barehanded without incurring sharp pain. Also, if my attention wanders toward a nettle plant which is not the one directly before me to gather, and I suddenly grasp it, I will get stung on the soft underside of my wrists. Gathering nettle constantly teaches me to be patient, to follow each small step right before me along my path in order to most painlessly reach the heart of my desires.

The prick of stinging nettle is in itself beneficial. The stingers contain histamines, acetylcholine, and formic acid, and the practice of striking the skin with a stalk of raw nettle (urtication) to bring blood to the surface of the skin and heat to rheumatic limbs has been used for centuries. Lore reports that the Romans brought nettle to England upon hearing Brittania's climate was cold; they intended to whack themselves with bunches of the leaves to increase circulation. The pain and itch of nettle sting is eased by fresh nettle juice, and by crushed violet, burdock, or yellow dock leaves. The liquid in the stems of jewel weed, my favorite poison ivy remedy, is also effective for easing the heat and pain of nettle venom.

Once, while sitting in my garden, I was approached by an old Slavic woman, bent sideways and walking with a cane, who pointed a trembling finger at my nettle patch. "This is the first time I see this in your country," she said. In her family they had used raw nettles to scour dishes as well as to heal arthritic hands by brushing the leaves over the joints. The sting of nettle eases the pain of sciatica, clears congestion in the muscles and lymphatic system, and warms cold feet. If you feel hesitant about flogging yourself, invite a bold friend!

Nettle can be used to regenerate damaged kidney tissue and to heal all maladies of the urinary tract, from stones to scanty urine, from incontinence to chronic cystitis. Regular use of nettle infusion will decrease one's desire for coffee and rebuild adrenal glands stressed by the consumption of coffee. I always recommend nettle to those who have a history of kidney failure and kidney-related diseases in their family. Nettle has been used to prevent the need for dialysis, assist diabetics, and to balance sugar levels in the blood.

Nettle likes to grow in nitrogen-rich soil, and feeds nitrogen back into the soil as well. The plant is rich in iron, calcium, magnesium, the vitamin B complex, vitamin K, and chlorophyll. Its vitamin and mineral content makes nettle a blood-building herb for those recovering from anemia and malnutrition, and is excellent for those whose faces are the color of chalk. Nettle infusion keeps the blood of pregnant women iron- and mineral-rich and is especially supportive during the last trimester of pregnancy.

Cooked nettle and nettle infusion enriches the quality and quantity of breast milk in humans and animals. Nettle strengthens the body after surgery, and the presence of vitamin K in the plant makes it an antihemorrhage herb, facilitating the clotting of blood, and slowing profuse menses.

Nettle is described, in many herbals, as eliminating fatigue and exhaustion. This is due to its blood-building vitamin and mineral richness and its effect on the adrenals and kidneys, which in Chinese medicine regulate the chi (life force) in the body. Nettle restores strength postoperatively and rebuilds the immune system, making the infusion and boiled leaves a wise ally for those living with HIV, AIDS, or chronic fatigue syndrome. Nettle can be given to children whose immune systems have been weakened by the overuse of antibiotics or vaccination. For children not ready for the chlorophyll-rich taste of nettle, a light infusion can be made and a pinch of mint added to the brew.

Nettle also benefits the respiratory tract. Its gently astringent leaves dry up coughs and strengthen the lung's ability to filter environmental pollutants. Children's coughs respond quickly to frequent small cups of strong nettle infusion and doses of fresh nettle extract. Cooking the young fresh leaves with barley and eating the porridge will unhinge deep bronchial congestion. Regular use of nettle infusion lessens the strength and frequency of allergies and hay fever and is a wonderful ally for those with asthma. The dried leaves can be burned and the smoke inhaled for easing tight lungs.

Long-term use of nettle infusion, or sipping nettle seeds steeped in wine, will add luster to one's hair and a glow to the skin. Infused nettle-seed oil will nourish hair growth and lessen dandruff. Nettle seeds have been used to nourish the thyroid gland and to reduce goiters. Herbalist Maria Treben reverently attributes to nettle the ability to prevent malignant growths over the course of one's life, and to dissolve cancerous growths in the stomach.

Nettle stalks are highly fibrous, and were used in western Europe and among the Native Americans to fashion clothes and nets for fishing. The high fiber content also hints at nettle's effect on digestion; regular use of the infusion invigorates the liver, gall bladder, and spleen, and acts as a gentle laxative, particularly if sipped warm in the morning.

Stinging nettle receives generous attention in the stories of Hans Christian Andersen, most notably in the story of the eleven swans. Princess Elisa endures the sting of nettle in order to spin yarn out of the plant's fibers and knit shirts for her eleven brothers, who have been turned into swans by their evil stepmother. She must stay mute until she finishes her work, casting the shirts over her brothers' swan forms, saving them only moments before she is about to be burned as a witch for her strange behavior. I love nettle's role in the fairy tale because it beautifully illustrates the weed's downright magical ability to positively transform whatever it touches. This herb is deeply alterative, steadily restoring vitality, energy, and health to all who honor her presence.

e⌇ NETTLE HAIR LOTION

1 qt of nettle infusion
¼ cup of vinegar
several drops of your favorite essential oil

When the infusion is ready, strain out the nettles. Add the vinegar and essential oil. I like rose, myself. Pour over towel-dried hair after shampooing and leave in.

e⌇ NETTLE GOMASIO

½ cup nettle seeds
½ cup sesame seeds
½ cup milk thistle seeds
¼ cup raw sea salt

The classic *gomasio* of macrobiotic cooking is a condiment made by toasting sesame seeds and sifting with sea salt. This recipe combines the calcium richness of sesame seeds with the kidney- and endocrine-toning effect of the nettle and the deep liver-regenerating power of the milk thistle. In a cast-iron pan, lightly roast all the seeds, then add to the salt and mix well. Lightly bruise the mixture in a mortar and pestle and sprinkle liberally over salads and in soups.

❧ SPRING NETTLES

4 cups of 6-8" tall nettles, cut
boiled water
organic butter
1 diced onion
garlic
olive oil
salt and pepper to taste

If you want to ease arthritic joints, go barehanded. Otherwise, with gloves, scissors, and basket, approach the nettle patch. Look for the tallest plant, and ask for permission to gather. Then snip the slender-stemmed plants. If the patch is large, gather the uppermost, or *aerial* leaves, leaving most of the stalk intact.

At home, cover the leaves with water. Bring to a boil and cook over medium heat for twenty minutes. This will tame the nettle stingers. The leaves will stay deep green over the whole cooking time because of the chlorophyll richness of the plant. Five minutes before the leaves are ready, sauté the onions and garlic in the olive oil. When the nettles are cooked, chop the leaves and add to the onions and garlic, just to bathe the leaves in oil, and evenly mix in the onions. Add salt and pepper to taste, and serve with a bit of butter on the tops of the leaves.

In some areas, the young nettles are tall enough to gather for boiling by mid-March. Harvesting the tops will encourage the stalks to grow new, tender leaves, allowing you to use fresh-picked nettle as a pot-herb through the end of May, when the plants begin to flower. Nettle gives forth both male and female flowers on the same plant, and their pollination habit is quite notable. As the male flowers uncoil, they fling their pollen into the air to be caught by the females, who produce the nettle seed. The play of the male and female nettle flowers is an imaginative expression of the fertility and partnership of the god and goddess revered at the May Day festival.

HAWTHORN *(Craetagus oxyacantha)*

At the old Beltane rites, a woman and man were chosen as the May queen and king to represent this marriage of the goddess and god. They were cloaked in green and crowned in wreaths twined of hawthorn blossoms, for the aphrodisiac scent of the flowers encouraged the couple to emulate the lord and the lady of summer by making merry in the fields all night long.

Throughout western Europe, the hawthorn is greatly esteemed as a magical tree bearing protective and visionary powers in addition to its renown amongst herbalists as a heart-healer. The *haw* in hawthorn means hedge, as the thorny-branched trees, which attain a height of thirty feet, were planted as hedgerows to effectively separate fields, the inch-long thorns preventing grazing animals from passing into a neighbor's meadow. Come fall, the creamy hawthorn blossoms of May transform into clusters of ruby-red berries, the waxy leaves turning crimson before they drop off the gray limbs of the tree. Come the early snows, the red fruits that dangle from hawthorn's spiked, bare branches glow like the cheeks of a child playing outdoors in freezing weather.

In Celtic tradition, it was believed that a hawthorn found growing with oak and ash was a sacred place where fairies dwelled, and that if one slept under the hawthorn at the full moon in May or on May Eve, one would behold the entrance into the land of the fairies. Hawthorn's association with portals has earned it a magical reputation as carrier of the power of the hinge, opening that which is shut, and shutting that which is open, as the tree deems fit. In Ireland, it was considered a grave act to hew down a hawthorn, for by felling the tree one lost the grace of its protective power over property, home, and family.

The wood of the hawthorn is fine-grained and suited for carving delicate items and magical objects. Charcoal made from its wood produced an extraordinarily hot fire; the ancient Teutons burned hawthorn branches on funeral pyres, believing that the souls of the dead escaped via the burning thorns. To this day, on May Day, travelers hang bits of clothing or ribbons in the thorns of this holy tree, murmuring wishes into the cloth. When shaken by the wind, these strips whisper the wishes into the ears of fairies prepared to whimsically bestow gifts upon humans. Like many relatives in the rose family, hawthorn is used in love spells: "charm of rose and hawthorn tree, bring my true love unto me."

Hawthorn's particular gift is as a cardiotonic. The flowers, leaves, and berries all have a nourishing, strengthening effect on the functioning of the heart muscle and on blood circulation. Hawthorn leaf, blossom, and berry extracted into water or spirit based preparations (recipe in October chapter) is a fierce, protective ally for those seeking to prevent heart-related conditions which are passed on from generation to generation. Used over a period of several months, hawthorn balances blood pressure by working in an amphoteric fashion; the flowers, berries, and leaves raise or lower blood pressure according to what is needed. Hawthorn assesses the state of the circulatory system and makes the necessary adjustments, restoring a steady cadence to the heartbeat, and smoothing out the flow of blood.

Consistent use of hawthorn extract elasticizes veins and arteries, dissolves plaque in these pathways, and increases the contractility of the heart muscle for more efficient pumping of the blood. Hawthorn eases heart murmurs, moves blood clots, and assists peripheral vasodilation. The plant is particularly helpful for those working with the challenges of heart disease. Used consistently several times a day for six to nine months as a tonic, hawthorn eases fluid build-up in the heart, decreases valvular insufficiency, and shrinks an enlarged heart. The berry extract calms a too-rapid heartbeat, soothes inflamed heart muscle, halts fatty degeneration of the heart, and aids those working with angina. Used at ten-minute intervals, hawthorn can dilate the coronary arteries.

Though powerful, hawthorn acts gently in the body. The medicine of this tree can be used safely by those taking allopathic heart medication. I have seen hawthorn, in conjunction with lifestyle and dietary changes, give people the opportunity to safely lessen and in some cases give up heart medication. Because the factors which contribute to heart disease are often related to lifestyle, diet, rest, and stress patterns, it is wise to consult a health professional and create a personally designed, multifaceted protocol for working with heart conditions. Sitting with the hawthorn tree or drinking the flower, leaf, or berry infusion helps us align with the heartbeat of the earth.

Gathered in the fall and steeped in brandy, hawthorn berries make a wonderful holiday cordial which warms the heart and increases circulation. The fruits can be used in the prevention of miscarriage, and a poultice of the leaves and fruits can draw out embedded thorns and splinters from the paws of animals. The berries, rich in vitamin A and C, also strengthen appetite and digestion, calm nerves, and ease insomnia. I sometimes use hawthorn to restore the strength of the heart following bouts of tonsillitis, strep infections, or rheumatic fever, which are known to weaken the heart muscle.

One need not be experiencing heart distress to benefit from the gifts of hawthorn. I often sip a bit of hawthorn berry brandy when my fingers and toes have gone numb with cold, or I need a bit of help in feeling warmhearted. As the guardian of the hinge, hawthorn wisely discerns the right timing for the wounded heart to open. Hawthorn berries and blossoms can be used to ease the grief of a broken heart and to open the heart to new love.

ℰ HAWTHORN BERRY BRANDY

handfuls of hawthorn berries
a good brandy
a jar

Wait until after the first frost, so the berries take on their deep red hue. When gathering hawthorn berries, one absolutely must leave a gift for the fairies, since one is gathering from a tree particularly sacred to them. After your first year of making brandy, you can leave a bit of brandy by the base of the tree or in one of its hollows for the spirits to sip.

After you have gathered the berries, place them whole, in your jar, and fill the jar to the top with brandy. Label the top of the jar with the date six weeks from now and wait. After the six weeks, you will have a tonic brandy that goes straight to the heart, and you will have a suitable holiday gift for all your friends.

ℰ HAWTHORN BLOSSOM BRANDY

hawthorne blossoms
brandy
a jar

No need to wait till winter for some heart-toning cordial. On May Day, gather the blossoms, and follow the directions as above for steeping. The flower brandy acts as an aphrodisiac and general producer of mirth and gaiety, the spirit of May, in addition to its heart-toning quality. I like to pass out this brandy on the summer solstice in June, which is about when the brandy will be ready for drinking.

The energies of hawthorn berry and blossom brandy are rendered distinctive by the seasons in which they are made. The blossom brandy holds within it the opening, fertile energy of spring as well as a lightness and gaiety carried within its flowers. The berries, as keepers of the hawthorn seed, hold the grounding, warming energy needed to shelter the seeds as the weather chills. As the flesh of the berries protect the reproductive seed of hawthorn, so the energy of protection is passed along to us through the berry brandy. When choosing between blossom or berry brandy, it is wise to discern whether the opening or protective energy is needed in relation to the person's spirit heart.

OPENING

In May, the gathering intensity of the sun saturates the plants and trees. The young, light green leaves on the tips of the maple and yew branches quiver in the gentle wind while the older leaves cloak the earth in a thick, forest green. The call of the birds becomes a daily background hum which invites our hearts to flutter in freedom and anticipation of the summer months. The deepening color and growing resiliency of the leaves in May carry within them a strength and maturity which become ours as we eat the wholesome gifts of the earth at this time.

As spring grows full, the plants and trees respond to the care given them by our efforts combined with those of the sun, clouds and rain by bursting into bloom. Early in the month, flowers adorn the apple and plum trees, scattering their petals over the ground, their fragrance wafting up to welcome the warm weather. Nature captures our attention, extending her pleasure-loving arms to us and opening her hand, finger by finger, revealing one profound flower treasure after another.

Flowers lure us into the present moment by the miracle of their beauty. Watching and waiting for a particular plant to bloom gives birth to patience within us. We slow our rhythm down in order to fully experience the process of flowering; expectancy and excitement deepen hand in hand with our patience. As we observe, we come to see that the full unfolding of the flower petals is the culmination of an unhurried dance in which the flower senses and responds, moment by moment, to the environmental conditions which surround and penetrate it. These conditions include temperature, moisture, light, and shadow as well as the more subtle influences of sound vibrations, heartful care, and respect.

In Buddhist poetry, there is a verse which reads: "I entrust myself to the earth, the earth entrusts herself to me." To entrust is to place something in another's hands with the confidence that what has been given will be cared for. For the thousands of years that humans have placed our trust in the earth, the earth has responded with abundance and grace, caring for us and delighting us with much nurture and beauty. However, in the past several hundred years, we have forgotten that the earth entrusts herself to us as well. We are learning that humans have a deep interdependent relationship with the earth and that when we do not care for the earth and tend to her with sensitivity and respect, we suffer in our mental, physical, and emotional well-being. Put simply, when the health of the earth deteriorates, our own health becomes fragmented.

Fortunately, our interconnectedness with the earth can help us reverse this depletion. Applying an attitude of care toward ourselves, as if we were the body of the earth, can greatly refresh both our spirits and the health of the planet we walk upon. We can work with May's blossoms in a way which gives us the necessary openheartedness to fulfill our task as trusted stewards of life on earth.

Wildflowers are keepers of joy. Resting our eyes upon them quickly elicits joy from within us, and so wildflowers are a bridge we can cross toward joy anytime we feel irritated or depleted. Flowers also exist inside our bodies in the form of joy. As Thich Nhat Hanh, Vietnamese Buddhist monk, notes, when we express joy through our eyes, our eyes become flower petals. When we smile, our mouths become blossoms. When we use our hands to comfort, to give love and care, our palms bloom. When we sing or laugh, we open the flower that exists in the heart and throat. The physical heart and womb especially, are delicate flowers that grow strong and open with our tender treatment and wither easily when treated with harshness. Indeed, the whole human body is like a flower, deeply responsive to environmental conditions and loving attention.

When anxiety, worry, and physical or emotional pain visit us, we lose our connection with the flower of joy that exists within us, and we often feel wilted. When this disconnection occurs, we are more likely to become unmindful; we may trample on other humans and on the earth as well. When we use the flowers as reminders to refresh ourselves and to reconnect with joy, we open areas of the body that have contracted in fear, returning to the birthright of our own rhythms as well as the rhythm of the earth.

On a fine day this month (of which there may be many), head outdoors with a basket, a small knife, or some scissors. Wear a hat to guard yourself from too much sun and pack a tasty lunch to take along. You may invite a friend, perhaps a young one, or an animal, to accompany you. Search out a garden or arrange a visit to a wild field filled with flowers you can freely pick from. You may choose a field of high grasses and reeds beside a pond, or a hilltop where the flowers are plentiful and low to the ground. Particularly for those of us who live in cities, seeking out and finding the small edens which exist in the midst of modern life can provide us with a steady source of refreshment throughout the year. When you find your spot, drink in the vista of the field, the play of light and wind on the plants and flowers, the sound of the bending grasses. Listen for the drone of the bees and other insects as they alight from flower to flower, gathering pollen.

If you feel comfortable, sit or lie down in the field you have chosen and let your body be warmed by the sun, your weight supported by the earth. Take two large blooms and place them over your eyelids and on your heart, peering at the world through your flower-laden eyes. Let your body open and relax to the heat of the sun and the pliant softness of the ground, recalling your innate sensuality. Listen for the voices of the fairy folk underneath the drone of bees.

When you feel ready, gather as many flowers as you can, choosing ones that are not yet fully unfolded, filling your arms with as much as you can hold as you wade through the grasses and pluck. Adorn yourself with sprigs tucked behind your ears, into your sleeves and neckline. Stand tall and inhale the intoxicating scent of wildflowers, relishing the bounty of color, the shapeliness of each blossom, the profusion of tiny and large blooms. Be aware of how alive and open the body becomes when it can welcome the sensations that compose its surrounding environment.

When you are satisfied, return home, creating bouquets of wildflowers for each room and adding them to the bath. Set aside some single flowers, pressing them between the pages of books you know you'll be reading while snuggled under blankets in winter. I love coming upon these tissue-thin petals when the trees are bare and I am curled up with a novel and a cup of tea. Beholding their flattened racemes and stems makes my heart flicker in reminder of the sumptuousness of late spring and brings a smile to my lips, for I know the season of fertility will return, again and again, my whole life long, filling me with that craving to open and feel the full beauty of the earth.

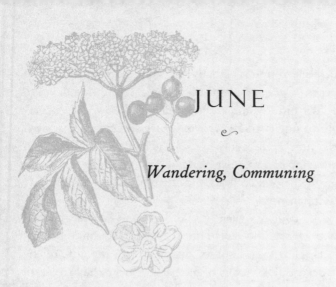

JUNE

Wandering, Communing

COME JUNE, THE sun unleashes a penetrating heat that liberates our bodies from the need for veils of clothing to separate our skin from direct communion with the elements. Now we can clasp the summer close to us, as one would a precious lover. The light of day unwinds and lengthens like an awakening cat and the earth frees her lushness under the bright gaze of our closest star. Crows pierce the mauve shadows of the fading night with their early cries to the dawn, and the sun settles its orange sphere into the horizon at a late hour. On the summer solstice, the daylight expands to its limit as the strength and vigor of the sun god, Lord of the Waxing Year, peaks.

When I was a small child I often flung myself outdoors, the screen door slamming behind me, insisting to my protesting elders that the solemn activities of the plant and insect world in June would not occur unless I gave my audience to them. There were butterflies and moths to be chased from yard to yard, the bright or earthy map of their wings fully contemplated. The bees needed to be watched as they hovered above the peony and rose bushes, diving into the inmost center of the flowers, their bodies wriggling as they wrapped their hind legs with pollen.

And then there were the mysterious egg sacs which my dad hid, in May, in the more secluded areas of the garden, threading these bone colored pouches to the branches of low bushes, out of the reach of robins, pigeons, and squirrels. In June, at exactly the right moment, these sacs exploded in hundreds of praying mantises, which clung upside down to the outer walls of their birth-womb and then dropped down, disappearing into the jungle of our Brooklyn lawn. These insects were so well camouflaged amidst June's green grasses that one had to train the eye to catch the sudden swaying of a singular blade of grass and raise one's eyes up the stalk to identify the cocked head, wide mandible, and supplicating forelegs of the praying mantis.

And then there was twilight, when hues of lapis and lavender melted the edges of concrete objects and pulled unearthly shapes from the deepening shadows. Bats, ghosts, and spirits emerged from the attic of the garage, from the stuccoed, back walls of the garden, from the bald earth behind the trunk of the Japanese maple as the talk of the night insects began. The rub of katydid wings yielded a rhythmic song which stilled the soaring flight of my young mind.

Legs dangling over the side of the back porch, I tucked my hands under me, palms warmed by the sun-baked flagstones, gaze poised for the floating light of fireflies. I waited. My breath rose into the quiet as the summer wind sighed into my ear and laid her cheek on the nape of my neck. And when they came, it seemed to me the fireflies used the lanterns of their bodies as a signal, for now the night fully descended and the stars began to grace the sky with their white lights. Relieved of my watch by the constellations, I rose and went inside, the screen door hissing shut behind me.

WANDERING

The freedom of my early years came to a screeching halt as I entered the first grade. The notion of nature as schoolroom had not yet become fashionable, and my need to explore the outdoors was severely curtailed as I learned while seated at a desk. In the midst of many lessons my attention was pulled beyond the windows by the sound of the wind swaying through the maples, and as summer came close, I began to almost writhe in my chair, certain I could hear the roar of the ocean calling me, though I lived miles from the beach.

During the week, my communion with forests and animals became confined to the books I swallowed whole, which described mansions surrounded by wrought-iron fences, covered in climbing wild wisteria, and rambling houses where ravens perched on the gables and toads lived in ponds hidden by willows. My mind perfected the magical art of being in two places at once; one part of me stored the rote, linear information I was gaining in the classroom while another part of me walked aimlessly through fields of heather and gorse in the moors of Scotland.

I had time for substantial roaming only on the Sabbath, when I could not do any writing homework. Though my territory became limited to the radius of one square Brooklyn block, I still found my heaven on earth: a forgotten plot of dirt which nestled between our neighbor's garage and the garage of our Italian friends. We had to dive into and part the thick vines of honeysuckle which concealed the area and then tear ourselves from the tangled branches to emerge, scratched but delighted, into our hidden grove. We came to call our gravesize hideout the "secretway," because we could slip around the corner to our playmate's house in just thirty seconds, instead of having to walk the whole block and risk encountering an adult who might restrict our play.

This spot became my wishing well. When I wanted to be lost, I would tiptoe out of the house, disappear behind my neighbor's garage, and untangle the honeysuckles, sipping their nectar as I took a wide step into the passageway, enduring surface wounds for the sake of being incommunicado. The telephone lines passed right over the secretway, and blue jays often perched on the wires and sat in vigil with me, breaking the cloak of silence with their occasional cries. The mound of earth I sat upon was filled with a few nail-ridden boards and flecked with chips of mica that glistened like diamonds, spurring my imagination to look for treasure. I plunged my hands into the soil and dug for riches, leaving the responsibilities of the mundane world behind me. I imagined that the yellow and white flowers of the honeysuckles were the gold and silver trumpets of fairies, who guarded me as I asked the imaginary inhabitants of this hidden home to fill my heart and restore a sense of peace within me.

By the time I was ten, I began to dress for fashion rather than for weather; I painted my lips and cheeks, combed my eyelashes with mascara, and slipped on high heels which crowded my toes and thickened my calf muscles. When the soles of my feet no longer had regular contact with the ground my body lost its connection to the earth. I came to fear the outdoors, to feel annoyed rather than awed by the weather, and to feel timid in the direct presence of the elements. The butterflies and fireflies were forgotten, the secretway left unvisited.

By the time I moved upstate for college, I had been almost thoroughly tamed. But some tiny vestige of my childlike wandering nature gave me courage to venture away from my home to a whole new environment. The sun god must have sung sweet songs of fertility to the land in Ithaca, for wherever one set one's eyes, there was the body of the goddess, rounded into the form of hills, dripping with waterfalls, glowing with red sunsets, and heaving up winter storms. In Ithaca, the elements were sovereign; by June during my first year of school I began to shed all the accessories which had walled me away from nature and returned my body to the earth, water, fire, and air. The soles of my feet began to remember their origins and I walked barefoot through the fall, my heart healed by the brilliant colors of trees, my heels slowly settling into the ground. When I grew cold, I warmed myself by hearth fires. When I was hot, I immersed myself in the gentle waterfall pools hidden in Ithaca's valleys.

I had no desire to return to the city. Come summer I stayed in Ithaca and lived in a room of many windows which overlooked the hills. Each morning I walked to Potter's Falls, where I let my body relax into the arms of the hot gray stones. In late afternoon I hiked the five miles home through the woods, following either the low path which ran beside the creek or the upper path which dipped and rose with the crest of the ridge. I picked Queen Anne's lace and dame's rocket, humming with the bees as I filled my arms with flowers.

Bending to pick blossoms, wading through shallow pools, I could feel the fullness of my female body like the body of the earth goddess. Away from the hungry eyes of men, I stretched my proud spine to its full height. I walked the five-mile length of land often, in all weather, keening my senses to the activity of snakes, toads, deer, and trees on rainy and cloud-filled days. I came to recognize the place of each stone, tree, and being that lived in the area, and my own place within, rather than apart from this sacred terrain. As I ambled without the judgment and voices of humans, my spirit came to roost like a bird in the serene home of my body. I became fearless in my wandering, and I felt free.

That summer in Ithaca was the first of many experiences in which the healing power of the elements enabled me to touch the home inside myself. The arrival of summer this month gives us the opportunity to wander out into nature, to forest, ocean, river, or mountain top and to return to the most liberated, soaring aspects of our selves. Janice Longboat, an herbalist and member of the turtle clan of the Mohawk, calls summer the season of fire, where we take care to keep the temperature of our body balanced since the heat of summer can be stressful on the heart. In traditional Chinese medicine, the season of summer is ruled by the organs of the heart and small intestine. Among their many gifts, the elder tree and lavender bush, which flower in the month of June, regulate temperature in the human body and lighten the spirit of the heart.

ELDER *(Sambucus nigra)*

The elder is considered a magical and holy tree by various cultures of western and northern Europe. Truly ancient, vestiges of her existence have been found at Stone Age sites. In Denmark, it was said that a dryad, called Hylde-Moer, the elder tree mother, dwelled in the branches of the tree and watched over it. If any part of the tree was cut without first beseeching the elder-mother, it was believed that she would haunt the family of those who had bypassed her consent until what was taken had been returned. In Copenhagen, the old sailor's section of Denmark, each house had a guardian elder tree and when one set out on a journey, the tree was entrusted with the health and safety of the traveler. If the tree remained vital, those within the house were certain the journeyer was safe.

It was believed that elder could not be struck by lightning, and so was planted nearby one's house. The stems of the elder branches, their pith removed, were worn as magical amulets to protect the wearer from harmful incidences and to bring health and good luck. Elderberries, blossoms, or leaves were hung over the doorways of houses in Russia to drive away spirits, serpents, and robbers, and one old magical chant hailed elder as an herb of prosperity: "elder over the doorway, fortune over the threshold." The bruised leaves were commonly used as an insect and fly repellent.

Blossoming at June's end, elder became woven into the rituals of the midsummer festivities, for its flowers fill the air with a pungent scent that causes drowsiness upon inhalation, its subtle narcotic effect giving rise to visions of fairyland. In Denmark, lore described that if one stood under the elder tree on midsummer's eve, one would behold the king and queen of fairyland riding by with a retinue of elves, nymphs, dwarfs, and other fair folk mounted on horses and playing pipes made of elder stems. In Irish fairy tales, it is said that the sidhe- or elf-arrows were fashioned of elder and that the most potent witch's wand was one formed from an elder bough. It was believed that the tree itself must grace the witch with a limb, and one was not permitted to cut a branch for this purpose.

Elder is considered the tree of transformation, guardian of the thirteenth month of the Celtic tree calendar. This month, which is three days long, contains both the end of the year, Samhain (Halloween) and the beginning of the New Year (All Soul's Day). The elder tree is home to the crone who carries many names besides Hylde-Moer: Calleich, Hel, Queen of the Underworld, and Freya, Norse keeper of the fire. This ancient goddess of many names who resides within the elder guards the doorway between the land of the living and the spirit realm of the ancestors.

Elder has been termed "the medicine chest of the country people." Its flowers, berries, and leaves all beneficially affect the body, as music emanating from pipes fashioned of its branches draws out the wood elves from the far glades to heal the spirit. Safe for even small children, an infusion of steeped elder flowers promotes sweating in order to regulate the temperature mechanism in the body. The presence of fever is an indication that the immune system is doing its work, and so elder may intensify a fever to bring it more quickly to a breaking point, or encourage heat to leave the body through diaphoresis.

Elder is often partnered with sweet-smelling linden blossom (*Tilia americana* or *cordata*), their combined diaphoretic ability drawing out excessive heat from the body. When inducing perspiration to bring down fever, it is vital that the person being treated lie in bed, wrapped comfortably in blankets, so he or she stays warm while the feverish heat leaves through the pores of the skin. Sipping the hot tea while soaking the feet or full body will induce perspiration, quicken the fever-reducing quality of the herbs, and bring calm and comfort to whoever is ailing.

Elder is the primary herb I use for working with flu. If I suspect that infection is present to a great degree, which a fever often indicates, I add echinacea extract, equal to half the person's body weight in *number* of drops, to the elder infusion. If heavy postnasal drip is present, I add yarrow flowers *(Achillea millefolium)*, which act as a wonderful astringent to inflamed sinuses and bring their disinfectant properties to the healing process. If the fever has dried out all the mucus membranes, I add comfrey or violet leaves to the concoction, their demulcent gifts restoring moisture to the system while increasing the expectorant activity begun by elder in the lungs. For very small babies, elder flower extract can be used to bring down fever, using a single drop per pound of body weight.

Elder flowers, soaked in water and applied to the face, lighten freckles and cool sunburned skin. Applied to closed eyelids, cold elder blossom tea rejuvenates eyes strained or worn by computer work, heavy reading, or squinting in the sun. Gypsies of medieval days refused to cut the elder for wood because of its miraculous ability to restore eyesight to those whose blindness had come from sudden shock. The leaves can also be soaked and applied to inflamed eyes. A salve made of the fresh flowers heals skin wounds, burns, and chapped hands. Fresh elder blossoms may be placed in a muslin bag and steeped in the bath water for a soak which soothes the nerves.

In August, the elder blossoms become blue-black berries which are edible and medicinal. The berries are rich in iron, and can be mashed and mixed with honey to make a quick, energy enhancing spread. The effect of elderberries is felt primarily in the lungs and in the digestive tract. The berries are mildly laxative, diuretic, and helpful in easing rheumatic pain. The dried berries can be used to ease diarrhea, and a necklace made of the hardened berries can be worn around an infant's neck and chewed upon to alleviate the pain of teething.

Like the elder flowers, elderberries can be used for coughs and colds; they bring up phlegm, alleviate bronchitis, and reduce fever. The berries ease tonsillitis and are used internally and externally for malignant skin growths. A syrup made from elderberries promotes the body's natural secretions and clears stuffed ears. Elderberry wine can be sipped for chills, flu, sore throat, and as an asthma remedy. Regular use of the wine clears the bone marrow and may help prevent cancers. The berries can be prepared as a vinegar for these purposes. Elderberries stuffed in dream pillows dispel insomnia.

Before I ever met the elder tree, I was taught that it carried the teaching of respect and relationship. Shortly thereafter, I was pleasantly surprised to find an elder tree right in my neighborhood garden. I was able to identify it by the characteristic, small, raised bumps on its flute-thin bark. For several years, I visited the tree on November 2, the Day of the Dead, and left a lit candle and some elderberry brandy for my relatives who had passed into the spirit world, as I asked for favors and listened for guidance. The small elder tree, unassuming beside the tall weeping willow, drew great attention in June, when the lazy, cream-colored flower heads covered the crown of the tree, which was only a foot taller than I.

Each time I gave a plant walk to the garden members, I explained how this tree teaches us of relationship: just as the blossoms and berries of this tree care for the health of the children, so must the elder generation care for the younger. That the spirit of the elder guards the safety of adults reminds us that the trees are our allies, and that it is our task, in kind, to protect the trees. The folklore around elder teaches us of the riches we receive when we respect the trees and the injuries, the "blindness" we incur when we neglect to revere them.

Within a year or two of my joining the garden and offering "weed walks," many mothers, communing with one another beneath the shade of the elder tree, learned of her profound skill in working with the health of children and regarded her with gratitude. Most went elsewhere to gather, since our garden held only this seven-foot high mother tree, and a single, three-foot tall baby. As the years passed, members came and left, the elder offering the secure, protective field of her energy to all who rested on the bench situated before her. One March, however, on one of my first wanderings into the garden to observe the early spring growth, I noticed something awry in the small area behind the bench. My heart sank. The two elder trees were gone. I looked closely at the bark of the sprouting shrub which had been put in its place. Though I found no raised bumps on this small plant, chills of anger began to prickle and raise the hair on my arms.

Over the course of several days, I asked many members if they knew what had become of the tree. Many gardeners were dismayed by its disappearance, and several people approached me, asking where the elder was. Finally, it became clear that two newer members had been given the common area (where the elders stood) to care for, and had mistakenly pulled out the elder. When I inquired as to the reason, one member replied that the tree was taken down because they hadn't liked the way it looked. I expressed my indignation, launching into a description of the medicine and lore of the tree. "Nothing I can do now," the member shrugged.

I walked away with my heart in my throat. *Nothing I can do now. Nothing I can do now*, repeated itself over and over in my head, growing in pitch to migraine size proportions. My need to give voice to my anger was so great that I had to take slow, deep breaths, and I slept fitfully that night, feeling justice for the beautiful elder must somehow prevail. But how?

For days I sat, wondering, sitting on the bench beneath the area gapingly empty of elder. It would not do to swallow my anger and accept this inequity, though that beloved tree was dead. I finally settled on writing a letter, stating how important the elder tree had been to the garden members. I decided to have as many people as I could sign the letter and ask that the garden vote, at the next meeting, to replace the tree. As the plan began to form within me, I felt more peaceful, and went to the garden to wade through the growing plants. As I passed the bench, I noticed the shrub was gone, and yet something else had been planted in its stead. I looked closely at the translucent green bark of this foot high plant. Raised bumps. I began to smile. Some magic far greater than mine had already been woven. We had a new, baby elder. Though there would be no blossoms this year, the protectress of our children had mysteriously returned.

I placed leaves from the rowan tree, the magical tree of protection, around the base of the elder, in the four directions, asking that the earth, water, fire, and air raise this tree to maturity. I scored a circle around the tree with the petals of blooming red roses. The news of the elder's homecoming quickly spread, and those of us who regarded the elder tree as a potent force were gladdened. Though I inquired, no one would claim having purchased a new tree. Several weeks later I found out that when the tree had been pulled, the roots had been left intact. The tree that appeared in the garden in June had actually sprouted from the original elder's roots, which were still embedded in the ground.

I myself have not always handled the plants mindfully. Shortly after my experience with the garden elder, I was out in the hills of the Catskills and spied a large elder in the distance. I picked my way through waist-high raspberry brambles to reach the tree, which was so tall I had to bend the branches down to pluck the flower heads. In my enthusiasm, haste, and desire to get the flowers, I forgot to greet the elder mother, nor did I ask her permission for gathering. I bent a branch down so quickly it broke off in my hands. Compassionately accepting my humanness in the situation reminded me to soften my judgment of those two garden members and of those who, in their ignorance, are awkward or hurtful to the plant world. Elder's skill in teaching about relationships was apparently at work here.

Celtic tree lore regards the elder as the tree of regeneration, representing "death in life and life in death." My relationship with the elder in the garden gave me a chance to experience the cyclical mystery of death and rebirth as well as the desire, flowing like a strong river within both my own being and the life force of the tree to adhere to this inner rhythm. The sense of serenity that settled within me with my decision to take action regarding the elder and the subsequent renewal of the tree imprinted in my consciousness the sensation of harmony which arises from following one's inner prompting and witnessing new life rise out of death.

ELDER FLOWER WATER

elder blossoms
½ gallon jar
boiled water
1½ ounces liquor (brandy, vodka)

When gathering elder blossoms, be sure to ask the spirit in the tree before picking. I like to gather the flowers on midsummer's eve, before the sun goes down, or on a full moon in June. Fill the jar completely with fresh elder blossoms and pour boiled water over them. Add the liquor and steep for several hours. Strain through cheesecloth and store in a pretty bottle.

Elder flower water can be used to refresh the skin, and as a magical potion for strengthening intuition.

ELDERBERRY CHUTNEY

1 lb fresh elderberries
honey to taste
1 small onion
4 ounces apple cider vinegar
ground ginger
cayenne
clove
mustard seed
sea salt

Mash the berries and mustard seed. Grate the onion. Mix together, adding honey, cloves, ginger, salt, and vinegar. Boil in a saucepan for ten minutes and let cool. Spread atop fragrant white rice, bread, or use as a condiment in sandwiches.

ℰ ELDERBERRY BRANDY

elderberries
brandy
jar with good lid

Steep the berries in the brandy for six weeks, adding some brandy every couple of days, to keep the jar filled to the brim. After six weeks, you will have a warming cordial which acts as a superb iron tonic while opening the sinuses and reducing fever.

ℰ ELDERBERRY SYRUP

1 ounce dried elderberries
1 quart jar
honey
brandy

Infuse the berries in boiled water for eight hours. Then heat two cups of the infusion under very low flame until you are left with one cup of decocted berries. Add several teaspoons of honey and a teaspoon of brandy to preserve the syrup. This syrup is an excellent expectorant.

ℰ DRIED ELDER FLOWER BATH

When gathering elder flowers, it is best to dry them on a screen. Treat the flowers gently, carefully placing the plucked blossoms in brown paper bags or a basket you can cover with a cloth, keeping the newly gathered blossoms out of the sun. If you can, have the screen suspended so that there is air below and above the flowers. Well-dried elder blossoms will retain their cream color, darkening to a slightly more yellow shade. If you buy elder blossoms in an herb store, make sure they are bone-colored and not brown. The blossoms can be stored either in a glass jar, away from sunlight and moisture, or in a brown paper bag.

To use elder blossoms in the bath, bind the blossoms in muslin or cheesecloth and tie to the nozzle directly in the flow of the bath water. The resultant bath will refresh the skin and relax the nerves, producing a mild diaphoretic effect.

ᘓ᛭ ELDER AND LINDEN FOOTBATH

1 ounce dried elder blossoms
1 ounce dried linden blossoms
quart pot
water

Bring the water to a boil. Add the blossoms and simmer for ten minutes. Sip tea of elder and linden as you soak your feet.

Most of us visit a physician to receive treatment when we injure our physical bodies, when we are confounded by the cause of our aches and pains, or alarmed by the sudden presence of unusual symptoms. The western medical model makes decisions about approach to bodily illness via diagnostic tools which quantify and measure disease. Homogenous standards of normalcy and health are set according to the limited range of experience which can be read by machines. The rich quilt of ancestry, gender, economics, culture, lifestyle, and life itself which creates physical variety and informs both health and illness defies categories and measurement. The nuances of wholeness slip through the fingers of finite, exclusively technical definition.

The foundational assumption of both tests and technological instrumentation is that the body can be described, viewed, and handled as a machine. This mentality has its roots in the Newtonian era, which seeded the ground of industrialism and laid the groundwork of our technological time. The Newtonian viewpoint placed the male at the center of the universe: both the earth and the human body were deemed inherently inanimate. Atoms were seen as inert, and the entire cosmos was believed to function as a machine rotating around a central male figure.

This philosophy, which outlawed our relationship with the earth as a sentient being, led to exploitation of the earth's resources and the degradation, exile, and attempted annihilation of all that carried mystery and wildness: nonhuman animals, trees, women, earth-connected cultures and traditions of healing. Newton's philosophy walked hand-in-hand with the Enlightenment era, which worshipped exclusively rational knowledge, gave birth to the art of war machinery, and placed all in service of the machine.

This philosophy, absent of almost any nutrition, has been empty food for our spirits, souls, and bodies. These values have affected our choices of what and how we create and destroy in all areas of our lives: religious ceremonies, forms of work, decisions regarding public and private space, education, our relationships with ourselves and other human and nonhuman beings, and our values. Viewing our health through the Newtonian lens has very nearly blinded our understanding of what causes both the deterioration and growth of wellness. Living under the false canopy of Newtonian-parts mentality, we have created a society which often undermines the spirit and muffles the soul.

The wounds which come from this form of injury do not show up on test results, which require us to administer to only the physical body. We often ignore the emotional component which diminishes or enhances our health, and indelicately omit nourishment and lifestyle transformations that unchain the soul and spirit as potent avenues toward restoring our physical well-being.

These invisible injuries often respond to invisible forms of healing: a comforting touch. A gentle, encouraging tone of voice. The scent of incense. The sweet juice of a fruit sliding down the throat when one is in despair. A song. The sound of a stream. A warm, sure hand lying over the hurt. A loving embrace. Glimpsing a flock of birds returning at winter's end. Giving someone a cool bath when she is burning hot. Offering water when one is feverish and bone dry. Opening a window in the sick room. There are as many forms of invisible healing as there are plants in the world.

The language of herbals of the pre-industrial era demonstrate an approach to health that appears to have been grounded in the understanding that bodily conditions were deeply connected to emotional well-being. There is an enormous canon of knowledge devoted to the tending of our emotional and spiritual ailments through the use of plants and foods, both internally and topically. Lavender is a wonderful example of a plant whose medicine quietly transforms the health of the body and the state of the mind.

LAVENDER *(Lavandula officinalis)*

Lavender's home is in on the western cliffs of the Mediterranean, but this plant has been cultivated extensively in France, England, and Australia. Simply gazing at its purple flowers, which bloom in June, causes a subtle but palpable lifting of the spirit. The upright spikes of the flower heads speak to the posture of attentiveness and revivification which is the human spirit's response to their scent and color. I think of lavender as the soft, substantial, and comforting hand of a caring human being which one can reach for while ailing. The effects of lavender are felt primarily in the nervous system and stomach, where the plant brings her soothing qualities. The light purple color of this plant indicates its affinity for the region of the brow and head.

Lavender has long been considered a woman's herb. For centuries it has been offered into the hands of women in labor: crushing the flower-filled sachets in their straining fists, the scent gives them courage and energy to continue the birthing process. Midwives also pass essential oil of lavender under the laboring woman's nose, or daub it on the temples to bring revivification to the taxed nervous system. This use leads me to believe the plant's emotional power is to give us courage when the path we are treading seems not only difficult, but highly painful. Courage can provide the momentum and support to help us cross emotionally stormy waters and lead us to the other shore.

Lavender is a grief-easing plant; it is an ally for those who have experienced loss of any kind, whether of a person, relationship, a vocation, or a part of the body. According to herbalist Rosemary Gladstar, lavender mixed with blue borage flowers are specific for lifting depression. Lavender as well as other "kitchen herbs" such as sage, rosemary, and thyme, are high in volatile oils which awaken the spirit dampened and immobilized by suffering. Like blue sky breaking through on a cloud-thick day, lavender brings renewed vitality and hope.

In the last century lavender was used to revive women prone to hysterical fits. The word *hysteria* comes from the latin word meaning womb; for women, the womb is the place where our instincts and deepest knowing of cycle and rhythm live. When a woman feels that her basic life force and freedom is somehow being compromised and she is not allowed to speak or act on her own behalf, she will often become hysterical. Hysteria is a self-protective response of the spirit, an alarm that a woman can learn to recognize within herself and act upon appropriately.

The difficulty with anxiety responses is that the strong emotions they produce often paralyze us or cause us to take ill-timed or ill-placed action. The life preserving emotions which accompany hysteria must be calmed before we can look deeply into the cause underlying anxiety and conceive of the fitting response. The scent and rich purple hue of lavender's blossoms inspire our sensuality, reminding us of beauty where there has been devastation. Lavender melts numbness, nourishing and keening our senses, the antennae of our instinctual knowing.

Inhaling a few drops of lavender essential oil revives those who have fainted, stills heart palpitations, and halts dizziness. The volatile, transformative passage of menopause, which often produces these symptoms, is greatly smoothed by the use of lavender. The popularity of this herb among grandmothers during and after the menopausal years is surely a sign of its potency and perfectly exemplifies invisible healing. The old wives' practice of burying lavender sachets in drawers, where the scent permeated one's clothes, or secretly carrying a bundle of lavender in one's pocket, allowed a woman to be bathed in its uplifting, steadying scent all day long while also preventing and easing menopausal giddiness and palpitations.

Lavender calms anxiety-produced headaches. Dream pillows scented with a single drop of essential lavender oil or stuffed with dried blossoms bring soothing, sweetening dreams and help one sleep soundly. Drops of essential oil can be added to footbaths to relieve tired feet, and can be used directly on the skin to ease the pain of second-degree burns. The essential oil diluted in a carrier oil can be rubbed on paralyzed limbs to stimulate them and to increase nerve power. The essential oil of lavender is *not* to be used internally. Lavender blossoms, wrapped in muslin and soaked in boiled water, can be applied to the joints to relieve rheumatic pain.

The practice of bathing in lavender was popular in Turkey and Egypt. The blue-purple flowers, infused in boiled water and added to the bath is my favorite way to melt stress and is recommended for women throughout pregnancy. I suggest that the bath be taken regularly by women raising children.

Lavender also acts gently on the digestive tract, where the dried blossoms prevent gas, relieve water retention, and halt digestive spasms. Fourteenth-century abbess Hildegard of Bingen used lavender as a tonic for the liver, boiling the flowers in wine and instructing the patient to drink little sips through the day for six to eight weeks. She mentions that this concoction also eases lung pain and clears steam in the chest and adds that this wine also provides a person with "pure knowledge and clear understanding."

Lavender also carries disinfectant and aromatic qualities which in the past made it popular in the swabbing of wounds, bruises, and bites and in the embalming of corpses. The steam of lavender uplifts the spirits of those in the sick room while clearing the air of infection. Sponge baths of lavender can be given to those who are confined to bed. The aroma of lavender keeps away flies and mosquitoes, and prevents moths. Lavender oil is effective in killing lice and parasites in animals. My favorite way to use lavender is to burn the dried flowers; the smoke imparts a sweet smell to the air and opens psychic vision. The stalks of lavender, divested of their flowers, were sold as straw and used for strewing the floors of churches. Wash the floors or walls in lavender infusion to magically cast out unwanted energies from the home and to restore a sacred dimension to one's environment.

I consider lavender to be a clarifying herb and an herb of beauty. It's effect is elemental, much like washing one's body in a clear stream after days of having no access to a bath. In the summer, I love to float the cooling blossoms in a bathroom sink filled with hot water and to cup the blue-tinged water in my hands as I bathe my face. Magically, lavender is used in spells for love, to draw sweetness and a mate who possesses both inner and outer beauty. The presence of lavender in the garden lightens the heart and invites us to return our gaze to beauty again and again.

ℯ LAVENDER HONEY

lavender blossoms and leaves
honey
jar

Fill the jar loosely with blossoms and leaves. Pour honey to cover, and let steep for six weeks. The resultant honey can be added to tea to soothe the nervous system, or can be taken in a ritual manner; while spreading the honey on bread, one can ask the lavender to spread sweetness throughout one's life. Lavender honey also assists one in having clear vision when one's mind is made murky by anxiety.

ℯ LAVENDER HEART SALVE

lavender blossoms and leaves
olive oil
jar
essential sandalwood oil

Follow the directions in the March chapter for making oil and salve. When the salve is still liquid and has been poured into small jars, add a single drop of essential sandalwood oil to each jar. This lovely salve is specific for rubbing on the heart when one is feeling grief.

ℰ LAVENDER FLOWER MIST

dried lavender blossoms
dried witch hazel bark
water
brandy

Place the lavender blossoms and just a bit of witch hazel bark in a saucepan. Put in enough water to cover the flowers, bring to a boil and then simmer for fifteen minutes. Turn off the heat source, and let the blossoms sit in the water overnight. In the morning, strain off the herbal matter, and add one part brandy to three parts lavender/witchhazel water. The solution should end up with 25 percent brandy to preserve the mixture. Place in a spray bottle and use for instant revitalization when hot or moody.

ℰ LAVENDER POWDER

dried lavender buds
1 cup of white or pink clay
1½ cups of cornstarch
lavender essential oil
muslin

In a deep bowl, whisk the clay and the cornstarch together. Start with one cup of cornstarch and add more as you like. The powder will take quite a few drops of essential oil. I tend to be on the cautious side, adding 3-5 drops and then waiting an hour to see how it sets. To add the dried lavender buds, grind them finely either in a mortar and pestle or a grinder purchased for the specific purpose of blending herbs and roots. Cover the bowl with muslin and let sit for several hours. Transfer to a spice jar with a shaker top or a pretty container.

ᕙ   LAVENDER BATH SALTS

equal parts: Epsom salts
> *borax*
> *sea salt*
> *lavender essential oil*

For this recipe you may use fine ground or coarse natural sea salt. Combine the salts and borax. Add just several drops of lavender oil and sift together. Let the salts sit for a while before deciding if you need more oil, as the smell of the lavender will increase after the mixture sits several hours.

COMMUNING

In June, as I wander through the thin aisles separating one plot from another in my community garden, the hundreds of flowers and aromatic herbs unique to each member's garden brush against my ankles, satisfying my soul's need to wade through flower-thick meadows. Each day I visit this changing place, inhaling the lavish scents and colors of blooming roses which open and fade throughout the month, my hungry eye always leading me toward some miraculous activity being engaged in by the birds, plants, and insects. Dozens of large, black-headed bumblebees alight on the flower heads of lavender, swaying on its thin spikes. Sparrows chase and swallow yellow jackets and the grapes plump out on the vine, shading the grape arbor with their cascading fruit.

The community garden of which I am a member is truly a testament to the transformative creative power of humanity. Originally an abandoned lot containing bricks from the crumbled foundation of an old building in New York City's East Village, several lone acres were nourished by a handful of dedicated people to become one of the most growth-filled areas of ground in Manhattan. I am astounded by the far-vision of these original gardeners, who were able to look at a trash-filled area and see the potential for thriving soil. The physical labor, the enduring efforts offered by these folk and the power of continuance inherent in nature joined to produce a sacred space of great beauty. Our garden has grown into a spirit-feeding touchstone for an entire ecological community: children, elders, cats, dogs, finches, wasps, and fruit trees all find food on this renewed land.

Mid-June, on a sultry evening, our garden hosts the great ladybug release. A clear glass box containing hundreds of ladybugs is opened and shaken over all the plots, the liberation of these creatures witnessed by many small children and their guardians. Overnight, the ladybugs are stirred out of the haze of their incubation. The presence of the ladybugs balances the population of aphids, insects that can quickly chew an overwhelming number of plants down to the ground. The morning after the ceremony, my walk through the garden witnesses a humorous scene of these red-winged, black speckled insects clustered together, often on top of one another, recovering from the shock of their liberation.

My daily walks through the garden arise out of my knowing that this little Eden helps me thrive. Wherever and whenever I walk slowly in nature and allow my mind to rest and my awareness to revive, the sight of lilies, birches, ferns, brooks, and spider webs seeps deeply into my inner soil, watering and feeding the place within me which grows, creates, dies back, and lies fallow according to the wise rhythms of earth. I call this place my inner garden; it carries my most fruitful dreams and visions and knows what I need to keep myself as verdant as the summer earth.

Particularly because the warm weather in June calls us outdoors, I find I can easily become overstimulated and lose my sense of this inner garden. I have taken to using lavender baths as a way to reconnect with the sacred terrain of my physical body, to be guided back before the secret entrance to my interior grove.

Sometime during June, gather lavender blossoms and dry the flowering stems, tying them with a colorful cord and hanging them upside down in a dry, cool place. If you have no access to fresh blossoms, buy a small lavender plant and keep it in a sunny window, or purchase the dried flowers, which are often available this month at the farmer's market or your local health food or herb store. When the flowers are dry, prepare a half gallon of the infusion and let it sit for several hours. Reserve some of the dried flowers for burning, hanging them in bundles over the bed or where the eye will catch them. The infusion can also be made with fresh flowers; when the buds lose their purple color, the liquid is strong enough for the bath.

When the infusion has sat for several hours, clear some time in your busy schedule so that you can fully enjoy your bath. It is best to take the bath at dawn or dusk, when the sky matches the color of lavender. I sometimes refrigerate my infusion and wait until I can find time to give my full attention to the bath. If I have refrigerated the infusion, I warm the liquid under a low flame as I fill the tub with bath water. While running the bath, prepare the bathing space: use either a shell or shallow bowl to burn some lavender blossoms in, and place that on the ledge of the tub, where you will be able to smell the smoke. Light a lavender colored candle, bathing the room in a soft light. Additional touches such as filling the room with flowers or playing calming music enhance the atmosphere. Keep a comfortable robe nearby which you can slip on as you leave the bath.

When the bath is ready, pour in the strained infusion. Unplug the phone and immerse yourself, soaking for at least fifteen minutes. Ignite the dried blossoms and watch the smoke rise, taking deep draughts of the sweetened air, giving lady lavender time to pull the strands of stress from your body, open up the brain to intuitive vision, and soothe the nervous system. Inhale the fragrant steam rising from the water, letting your cares drift away, settling completely into your body. Sense your body as the garden that it truly is.

When you step out of the bath, wrap yourself in a soft robe and rest. Let the soothing energy of the bath linger even as you walk out into the balmy June evening to watch the coming of night and the rising of the moon.

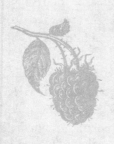

JULY

❧

Thriving

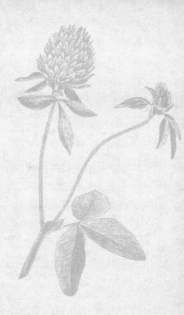

IN JULY THE jubilance of summer can be seen everywhere one turns the head and settles the eye. The abundant gifts of nature weigh down the branches of trees and offer themselves to us; squash blossoms lengthen into the first fleshy gourds, beans hang like earrings off vines, and tomatoes fatten, flashing their brilliant red and adorning our leafy salads with their seed-laden, juicy flesh. The creative zeal of the land finds its way into our kitchens, where we deepen this creativity with our mealmaking and preserve summer's ripe energy, captured in July's food plants, through canning, pickling, and wine-making. Nature's generosity at this time inspires us to extend our hospitality to friends and family and to celebrate the richness of the land.

By day, the sun's rays enter into fruits, vegetables, and flowers, and the air is filled with delicious scent. By night, July's alluring warmth calls all creatures out into a steamy atmosphere and star-filled sky. The temperature makes it possible for us to linger in the dark, to breathe in the patterns of the stars and the subtle glow of the moon. We can walk and watch, listen and float in the dark as the night creatures do, refining, like owls and bats, our night vision and aural ability. Moving about at night allows us to develop the skill of both becoming and interpreting shadows; we learn to step in light yet firm harmony with the creatures who move about within the veil of blackness. The temperature, approaching that of our blood when we are flushed with excitement, makes it possible for us to enter the darkness freely, our clothes thin enough for skin to directly receive the charge of the night air, which heartily enfolds us in its humid, salty embrace.

The Orthodox Jewish community in which I grew up, had ways which were given to them through the holy book, the Torah, as well as unwritten customs that were passed on through the centuries. Much as a cook sifts through grain to pick out stones, rabbinic scholars pored through the written tenets carefully, codifying certain ones and arguing heatedly about others. But behind both the laws and customs were the invisible structures and practices which kept the people together in quiet times as well as periods of great strife. These invisible cords were often woven not by the scholars, but the simple folk, ofttimes the women, in the invisible yet enduring manner which is the trademark of commonness.

One informal but potent habit of my neighborhood people was to stroll the summer streets after dark, ostensibly to walk off the heavy Shabbat meal. For the budding libido of a young woman or man, these walks were the most exciting of occasions, for one was never quite sure who one might stumble upon in the dark. Perhaps one would encounter the family whose handsome son was fancied by one's sister; older, more settled folk might have a chance to inquire into the health of a neighbor's elderly father or grandmother. The unannounced news of an engagement often passed from ear to ear in this manner.

At this time, due to particular Sabbath laws, families walked without carrying any books or bags, and were dressed in festive holiday clothes. The murmur of conversation surrounding each cluster of humans floating through the dark blended with the hum of night crickets. In the heat-heavy darkness, from a distance, I tried to guess the identities of the walkers by the shapes of the shadows moving toward me. I vividly remember one couple, close friends of the family, who often walked far behind their children. Whenever we ran into this pair, it seemed we caught them in the middle of a silent communion, their fingers laced together like spiders in close embrace. Though they were outwardly quiet, I had the feeling that they were speaking through their locked hands. The pace of their walk was unhurried, their footsteps slow and contented. Filled with the bounty and ease of summer, secure in their love for one another, their serenity settled over all in their wake: the air, the maples, and the children of other promenading families.

The strength of the sun and the humidity of the environment in July can press uncomfortably close to us, bringing home yet another comforting gift given to us by the plants and trees: shade and shelter from the unremitting gaze of the sun. When the mugginess becomes so heavy it seems even the air cannot carry it, clouds swell with moisture and collide, breaking open and showering the earth with torrents of water. The rains of July pull up a rich, loamy smell from the ground which makes us toe the earth and lift handfuls of dirt to our noses. While certain tender plants cannot withstand the sometimes sharp force of July's thunder-showers, the shifting tempo of rainfall causes great spurts of growth in the plant world.

For the food plants that are able to ride out the waves of heat and storm, the turning wheel of sun, heat, and rain hastens the ripening of tomatoes and brings first blush to green apples swelling in the orchards. Those who keep gardens or farm fields welcome the rainfall, so essential in bringing the greens, fruits, roots, and tubers to maturity. When we experience a summer either scant or empty of rain, the sun and heat scorch the green nations and drain the reservoirs of our own vitality.

When the heat reaches an intensity that pulls out our internal reservoir of moisture, it is to the water we turn, water which the earth has kindly caught in her hollows and kept ready for us. Whether we choose ocean, river, creek, or lake in which to cool our overheated bodies, it is the water in summer which is both precious and required for our survival and comfort. The rains refresh and revive the plants, a grass-green scent rising off the delighted, water-drenched leaves. In July, as we sink our heat-worn skins into cool and wet streams, we emerge sweetened and restored. How sacred is this water, whose renewing substance keeps the land, and all upon the land, lush, vibrant, and alive. Clearly, water is crucial for the growth and thriving of all earth's inhabitants.

THRIVING

In creation myths of many cultures, the source of all life is imagined as a vast, oceanic mother. Within the vessel of her body she contains, nurtures, and shapes the undeveloped forms of life within her watery womb and births them onto a land revealed as she recedes into her own dark mystery. Until quite recently, as we bathed in rivers, as we carried water from stream or well to home, humans had frequent sensuous intercourse with this fundamental source of life and thriving.

Today, few of us carry weighty ceramic jugs we have fashioned from clay and baked, to hold water hoisted upon our shoulders. The circumstance of receiving instantaneous comfort which is a boon of the twentieth century is made possible by an arena of technology which allows us to benefit from the earth's resources without, quite literally, having a hand in the gathering and directing of these resources. The immediate availability of even heated water from our faucets and showerheads allows us to easily disconnect from the source of this water and from the tidal ebb and flow which once kept us close to a cycle in which the currents coursed, at times strongly and at times lightly, down its oft-used paths.

Our separation from this source has been costly. Accustomed to the constant accessibility of water and physically removed from its taproot, we have caused this precious element to be polluted by the byproducts of our industrial creating. Our dumping has heavily poisoned the water, killing the diverse life forms that live within it, that feed us and are fed within its salt and freshwater environment. Because our bodies are microcosms of the earth's body, we are experiencing a rise in illnesses of the fluid-related and cycle-dependent areas of the body: the lymphatic system, the womb, the ovaries, and the prostate gland.

Ironically, what began as a perhaps well-meaning attempt to make water available for all has mutated into a complicated system of pathways which has not only literally cut us off from the actual wellsprings of our water but has also amputated us from a felt relationship to water as matrix, as mother, as womb of all life, as receiver of our pains and celebrations. Many of us are cut off from our primal mother in a way which leaves a dry emptiness we find difficult to name. The ascription of divinity to the elemental forces kept a sense of sacredness, power, and mystery intertwined with the idea of water as source. The simple, reverential manner in which we related to the cyclical ebb and flow of water nurtured a feeling of thriving and abundance within the spirit of each person.

Still, we can take heart. For while our connection to the elemental power of water has withered in this century, parching our instincts around nurture and revivification, the natural cycles of life, death, and rebirth remind us that our lifeline to this mystery and our ability to flourish can be recaptured. Though we may lose our course and our umbilical cord to our watery mother, the water—indeed none of the elements—ever forsakes us.

The drama of a summer thunderstorm gives us an opportunity to reacquaint ourselves, to become more intimate with the movement and language of the body we live on and places us in the heart of a natural event which recharges us and renews our connection with our source. Taking time to watch, listen to, and feel a thundershower is a simple practice which can begin to water seeds of passion for life within us.

All of nature announces the coming of a summer storm and makes way for this wild force to pass through. Dead leaves whirl in ascending spirals that follow the air currents; the wind courses through the reeds, pines, and birches which bow and bend to her power. The flight of gulls, pigeons, and sparrows are accompanied by urgent cries, spreading news of the approaching squall. Ground creatures make hasty preparation to shelter themselves, and the air fills with a palpable electrical charge as the light shifts to otherworldly hues. Human eyes turn skyward, watching and waiting for the breaking of this gathered power.

In the Native American Seneca tradition, the thunder, lightning, and earth are all seen as sentient beings which perform a mating dance whose purpose is to express love and to renew the energies of the Earth Mother. The sonorous rumble of the Sky God is his mating call to the earth. The low hanging, full-bellied, dark clouds are called the thunderbeings, and are seen as the many lovers who descend as raindrops to the Earth Mother to fill her with new energy. Rods of lightning, "fire sticks," are understood to be both the bridge between the Earth Mother and Sky Father, as well as the physical expression of their love for one another.

The magnetic field of the Earth Mother is greatly nourished by the electrical energies in the jagged bolts; the moisture in the sky becomes the Rain People, who descend to quench the thirst of the Earth Mother, that she will grow full enough to feed all growing things.

Thunderstorms are exciting; they raise energy and shower it over all beings, arousing us with their wild, almost sexual passion. My own heart still throbs at the approach of summer storms; as the wind shakes the trees and the light is jaundiced in the midst of the afternoon I am stricken by an impulsive desire to hurl myself into the storm's center. As a child, with the first rumble of thunder I ran out to the patio and unrolled the black and white striped awning to catch the rain. I sat beneath its canopy, watching crows and starlings balance on the swaying telephone lines. My skin quivered in response to the heightening wind as I dragged the rain-barrel out into the open to catch the falling water. Crawling under a blanket, my sister and I waited for the storm to break. We watched the sheets of rain and wondered if God really was crying, as mother had told us. Sometimes, the sun would emerge and illumine rainbows of light within the drops of water. If the sun came out, I felt emboldened to dance in the sheeting rain.

When the water stopped, we walked barefoot on the rain-drenched grass and kept watch for a possible rainbow. The abundance of water which fell from the sky amazed me, though part of my small child self already knew enough to fully understand how God could cry so many tears in a single day.

Whenever it rains, I say a blessing for the water which keeps my garden growing. We have all experienced years when rain has been slight during the spring, and the rivers, reservoirs, and streams seem noticeably low come summer. By being careful with the water we do use we become the nurturant water mother ourselves and care for the earth with the maternal tenderness she has given to us. If no summer rain arrives in July to break the weighty heat, then the trees will begin to show the frayed, brown leaves symptomatic of their discomfort.

Similarly, without the irrigation of July's thundershowers, we too dehydrate and shrivel. During summer, Hildegard of Bingen advised, we need to keep our bodies moist and juicy in order to thrive as all nature thrives. The herbs I have chosen for the month of July nourish the endocrine system, which tends to the secretions of the body, and in particular, to reproductive discomforts which arise from hormonal imbalance or injury to the soul of our reproductive sexual organs and lives. While these herbs are particularly useful for women, the glandular systems of men benefit as well from the simple power of these plants.

RED RASPBERRY *(Rubus idaeus)*

I once took a kindergarten class to our community garden for a wild edible walk. I spoke about a single herb, and was about to move on to another when one child spotted the ripe red berries hanging off the raspberry leaves. Within moments, the children had swarmed the small meadow where the raspberries lived and gave their complete attention to plucking berries. I quickly abandoned my plan to wander through the garden and discuss the wild green foods. These children had quite rooted themselves to the dwelling place of the raspberries and chosen their own wild food. I attempted, with mild success, to slow the children down and teach them how to respectfully pause, identify the largest presiding raspberry, and ask the thorny grandmother for permission to pluck the fruit of this wondrous bramble.

Raspberries are devoted to life and thriving. The sweet, cooling taste of wild raspberries reminds us to savor the pleasures of life; her thorns remind us to protect the joy in our lives from those who would pluck it from us, and to mind and tend to the abundance that has been given us. Closely watching the growth habits of the red raspberry reveals its medicine gifts. The berries on a red raspberry cane do not ripen at once; the appearance of the fruits seems timed by the plant itself to allow for picking them over the period of a fortnight. This intelligence of rhythmicity and timing suggests to me that in the human body, the plant might affect the hormonal system, which governs and nourishes rhythm.

Growing profusely in areas where humans tread, the bent canes of red raspberry echo the posture of the elderly, bowing earthward so that both child and small animal can taste of this plant's mouth-watering fruit. The thorns on the canes of red raspberry often hover over ground which has at some time been disturbed by careless human use. The brambles protect this ground, their thorns preventing humans and other animals from treading upon it, giving the soil space and time to regenerate.

Red raspberry is in the rose family. Its leaves usually grow in groups of three off the stem, and the backs of the leaves are silver white. The silver back of an herb often indicates its relationship with the moon; these plants usually affect the reproductive system and restore lunar rhythmicity to women who drink these teas. The configuration of three leaves, two pointing outward and one between them pointing down, mimics the position of the ovaries and womb. When chewing the leaves of this plant, the tongue and mouth become dry, signalling red raspberry's astringent quality.

Red raspberry is first and foremost an herb of fertility, pregnancy, and birth. Its leaves are rich in calcium, magnesium, vitamin C complex, thiamine, niacin, carotenes, and other trace minerals. The vitamin and mineral content of this herb make it a nutritive tonic to people of all ages and provide the body with nutrition that brings fertility and strength to both women and men. The infusion is a fine substitute for black tea, for the tannins in red raspberry lend a slightly bitter flavor to a brew prepared from its leaves which is similar to that popular beverage.

The plant contains an alkaloid known as fragrine, which strengthens the uterine and pelvic muscles. The high vitamin content of red raspberry unites with the power of fragrine to make it *the* herb of choice in preparing a woman's womb for pregnancy. Fragrine facilitates the birth process by toning the uterine muscle throughout the whole of a woman's pregnancy so that it more powerfully contracts and expands during labor.

During childbirth, mothers can suck on ice cubes of red raspberry leaf infusion to keep the contractions of the uterus rhythmic and strong, moving the labor process along. Red raspberry also helps bring down retained afterbirth and is often drunk by women throughout their pregnancies to prevent various difficulties unique to each trimester and to nourish the growing fetus. Sipped as an infusion in the months following the birth, red raspberry restores the elasticity of the womb and provides the new mother with nutrients that enrich and increase the flow of breast milk.

The thorny canes of raspberry simultaneously brandish flowers, leaves, and berries on the same bush, suggesting to me that this plant is useful for all cycles of life. Lover of children and elders, adolescents and adults, red raspberry is a powerful, gentle tonic for girls becoming women, for women seeking to become pregnant, and for men seeking greater fertility. Its leaves provide excellent nutrition and endocrine balance for those passing through the archway of girlhood to womanhood or through the menopausal passage. The calcium in the herb calms the nervous system and strengthens the hormonal system.

For a young woman, regular use of red raspberry leaf tea can establish a rhythmicity of menstruation which will serve her through the emotional torrents of adolescence. Like a midwife, red raspberry helps women ride smoothly through the sweeping changes of the menopausal years, assisting the transition as the woman gradually comes to hold the power of her monthly courses energetically within the womb. The carotene richness of the plant helps renew the blood sometimes lost by women who bleed profusely during the menopausal years, eases midcycle spotting, helps keep bones strong and flexible, and prevents brittleness. Red raspberry is often combined with other herbs, such as horsetail *(Equisetum arvense)* to aid in bone mending. The leaves can even be applied externally for prolapsed uterus.

Red raspberry works beautifully to restore menstrual cycles which have become irregular due to prolonged use of the birth control pill, the difficult and stressful experiences of miscarriage and abortion, or poor diet. For this purpose, a woman drinks several cups of the infusion daily for a fortnight each twenty-eight day moon cycle, either beginning on the full moon and pausing at the new moon, or beginning at the dark of the moon and drinking the infusion until the moon becomes full.

For some women this process brings back the menstrual flow quite quickly; for others, a year of use may be needed to gently and gradually balance the menstrual cycle. Restoring the link between the menstrual cycle and the phases of the moon often provides a profound homecoming for women that feels remembered rather than learned. The plant and the moon are used as allies to rekindle a sense of regard for the cyclical nature of our lives, for the tides of being and doing, of waxing and waning which occur within us on a monthly basis.

It is my belief that the pressure upon women and men to adhere to only one cycle—an outgoing one—and for women especially to perform business as usual during the sacred menstrual time contribute to the high incidence of reproductive difficulties, from heavy cramping to endometriosis to cystic and fibroid thickening. These difficulties tend to call us back to the womb, giving us the opportunity to repair our respect for this miraculous inner vessel which thickens with nurturant blood and releases this minerally abundant uterine lining back to nature each month.

In more ancient times, women often bled together, by the dark of the moon. They removed themselves from daily activity and went into lodges, determining the future of their community through visions received during this magical, potent time. Women gave their blood to the earth, or caught it in soft moss or animal skin they wore close to the vulval opening. Today, women are subtly or forthrightly asked to view this blood which nurtures new life as a "curse," and are encouraged to hide it, masking all signs of this sensitive and powerful time through drugs and other means, and to act as if we are of only one cycle. We learn to stop our natural flow, to catch it before it shows, to hide it or flush it quickly away.

I believe these attitudes contribute to heavy cramping and other dificulties women experience during the menstrual time. When a woman catches her blood in more natural materials, when she gives her blood to the elements in a proud, self-loving manner, and most importantly, when a woman can take solitude and replenish her inward flowing energy during this sacred time, the general health of her reproductive area increases.

Men are also subject to cycles, bound to the moon and sun in their own intimate, mysterious way. A culture which removes men from coming into contact with the life-nurturant, internal energy expressed by menstruation, that encourages men to adhere to a constantly outgoing cycle, greatly injures the inner life-loving, creative counterpart of the womb in men: the area of the prostate. The insistence that men hold in their tears often results in a backlash whereby emotional pain is thrust back into the watery, hidden recesses of the body. The current high incidence of prostate cancer may be an inner call for men to return to the needs of their own cycles, and to tend to their emotional lives.

Men too need to find ways to keep themselves moist, creative, and generative, returning to times of stillness as well as activity, and nurturing the seeds of respect for life and the desire to protect and preserve it which lives within them. According to herbalist Juliette Levy, wild raspberry foliage and shoots are a well-known tonic for stallions and bulls. To me this indicates that regular use of red raspberry leaf infusion can assist men in discovering their wild, sacred fertility.

Herbalist James Green echoes my belief that men benefit from reproductive herbs traditionally used for childbearing and menopausal women. He asserts that men are subject to a cyclical vulnerability and moodiness and receive little, if any, support in honoring the cyclical nature. He suggests that much like the menopausal woman, men pass through a "change of life" which allows them to mature emotionally, using this strength to develop patience, see clearly, and "step into the courtyard of functional wisdom, compassion and compromise." He recommends the use of red raspberry as a foundational herb for nurturing and maintaining hormonal, cyclical hardiness.

In addition to red raspberry's skill with the reproductive system, the astringency of its leaves ease diarrhea, particularly in the case of children. The tea soothes sore throat and the leaves, soaked in boiled water and chewed, can be applied to canker sores of the mouth, cooling, and tightening inflamed tissue. The calcium in the plant aids in building healthy bones and teeth, while red raspberry combined with other herbs dries out the excessive vaginal mucus often present in candidalike conditions.

Red raspberries provide iron and are an old folk remedy for anemia, paleness and worry. The fruit is a mild laxative. According to Mohawk herbalist Janice Longboat, raspberries are the "leader" of the summer fruits and cool the heart which can be taxed by summer's heat. Use iced red raspberry infusion in place of iced black tea, refreshing the body as much as a dip in the water.

℮ RED RASPBERRY POPS

red raspberry leaf infusion
organic apple juice
Tupperware popsicle trays

Gather red raspberry leaves which are not in flower. Dry them and make an infusion, following the general instructions in the March chapter, using two ounces of leaves per half gallon and steeping for four hours. Mix the infusion half and half with organic fruit juice and pour into popsicle trays. Put in the freezer, and the following day you and your loved ones can enjoy this cold, nutritious treat.

ᘓ WISE WOMAN/WISE MAN TEA

red raspberry leaves
nettle leaves
mugwort leaves
½ gallon jar
boiled water

In this concoction, red raspberry leaves strengthen the womb and prostate; nettle leaves toughen the spirit and provide energy and nutrition; and mugwort, the strongest tasting herb of this brew, eases cramping and stimulates dream activity and one's inner wisdom (see "November"). Adjust the amount of each herb according to the qualities you most want, using a total of two large handfuls in a one-half gallon jar and making an infusion. You can also use a teaspoon of each herb in a large mug, cover with boiled water, and steep the tea for ten minutes. The quick tea will not be as mineral rich as the infusion, but the quality of magic will still be felt.

This brew is best sipped hot, while wrapping oneself in soft blankets or shawls whose colors are evocative of the womb. Women can drink this tea during their moontime, men and women can sip the brew on the full or new moon, or whenever one needs to return to the deep nurture of solitude. I always drink this tea in the late evening and, if needed, ask the spirits for dreams of guidance. I keep a journal by my bed to record my dreams upon waking.

We sometimes minimize the deep effect that the food we take into our bodies has on not only our physical health, but also on our emotional and mental health. In the tradition of herbalism in which I apprenticed, I learned to recognize, by listening carefully to my body's cravings, which foods dampened my life force or quickened my desire for life. Long-term self-experimentation with nutritive herbs led me to the understanding that certain wild plants, often the ones we disdain and discard as "weeds" because of their persistent ability to thrive in challenging environments, act as food within the human body. The medicine of these plants tend the garden of the human body, lovingly and steadily enriching our soil, our cellular foundation in a way which ultimately alters the quality of every thing grown in this fecund ground. These ancient, wild foods, eaten in salads or dried and used as infusions are heartily welcomed and easily assimilated by the human body, causing no stress to any organs and greatly satisfying an omnipresent and lingering hunger caused by nutritionally empty food, vitamin-weak fruits and vegetables, or chemically laden meat.

During my herbal studies I also came to understand and view the human body as a living, changing being. Our cells are constantly being born and dying, often giving us ample opportunity to feed new cells with optimum nutrition and slowly shift the ground of our health to a state of vitality, regardless of age. Certain herbs, used as infusions and also as broths for soups, build and enhance the health of children, adults, and elders at the deepest level. Interestingly, most of these herbs tend to grow quite commonly and abundantly under our very feet, making them accessible to all. These herbs nourish the hormonal and nervous systems, triggering the release of chemicals which calm the mind and keep one's nerves able to withstand the stress of modern life. Red clover is such an herb.

RED CLOVER (*Trifolium pratense*)

Growing close to the ground, each sturdy pink flowerhead of this wild weed absorbs vitamins and many trace minerals from the earth beneath its three oval leaves. A member of the legume family, red clover, a European immigrant, contains the full chain of amino acids, making it a perfect protein easily absorbed by the human body. In addition to protein, red clover also contains calcium, vitamin B complex, thiamine, niacin, vitamin C, chromium, magnesium, nickel, potassium, and phosporus. As a vegetarian for over twenty years, I find red clover gives me strength when my blood sugar levels are beginning to tip due to lack of food, premenstrual hormonal swinging, and a need for protein.

Red clover is considered an alterative herb, possessing the ability to send its medicine into many areas of the body at once, providing deep and lasting change in chronically stubborn conditions. In addition to restoring smooth function of various organ systems, alterative herbs help the body assimilate nutrients and eliminate metabolic wastes. In general, alterative herbs are helpful in working with infection, blood toxicity, and skin eruptions. Red clover's alterative strengths are most directly experienced in the lungs, the nervous system, the lymphatic system and the hormonal system.

In the female body, red clover and red raspberry work together to enhance fertility. The strengthening of the uterine muscle is enhanced by the red raspberry; red clover balances the acid and alkaline levels, making the vaginal atmosphere conducive for successful fertilization of the ovum by the sperm. Optimum nutrition is provided by either fresh or dried red clover blossoms, strengthening the womb in preparation for the childbearing year. Its endocrine balancing properties nourish those glands which release the juices of sexual desire. Red clover does have a tendency to thin the blood, and so is best avoided when dealing with situations where blood loss is present, such as menopausal flooding, fibroid related bleeding, and heavy menstrual cycles.

Red clover can be drunk as an infusion when infection is present and the lymphatic system needs to be functioning optimally. The plant's diuretic quality is helpful in keeping fluids moving through the lymphatic channels, and is indicated when lumps or lymphatic swellings are present, particularly around the ear and throat area. An expectorant as well as antispasmodic, red clover is specifically indicated as a tea and syrup for easing dry, hacking coughs. Its affinity for the lymphatic system makes the plant a suitable building herb for those dealing with lymph-related cancers or conditions which require a strengthening of the immune system, such as AIDS, cancer and a variety of autoimmune diseases. Traditionally, red clover has been applied externally as both poultice and ointment and drunk internally to heal skin cancer. The plant is being used in cancer prevention, particularly as a tonic for men at risk for prostate cancer.

Sometimes referred to as a blood "purifier", red clover keeps the liver in healthy condition so that blood is well filtered. Soothing to the nervous system, draughts of infusion are greatly beneficial in times of high stress, applying a balm of fertility to the field which has been burnt to the ground, as in situations where one has lost the desire to live as the result of a traumatic, spirit-rending experience. Here red clover acts as a nurse to the child within who is often deeply wounded by injuries to the spirit. I imagine red clover as a healer who cups one hand behind the head of the ailing spirit child and brings a drink to their lips, each sweet sip renewing one's connection to life while cooling the inflamed edges of the nerves.

Infusion of the flowers is effective in relieving the pain of arthritis and is useful in providing relief of the sometimes intense pain related to rheumatoid arthritis, an autoimmune condition. The calcium in red clover, easily absorbed and used internally, supports the body in releasing calcifications caused by synthetic calcium, which tend to create pain around the joint site. It is an excellent herb for those suffering from terminal illnesses, who are weakened by the hospital experience and are confined to a diet of liquids. The infusion serves as a food, providing nourishment when the body's energy cannot be focused on digestion but is focused on general life support. Children love the sweet taste of red clover and develop strong immunity as a result of regular use. Mildly sedative, red clover is specifically indicated for inducing deep, healing sleep in children.

Magically, finding a two-leafed clover means a lover will come to you again. The four-leafed clover brings luck in whatever area the finder is lacking, be it love, wealth, health, or serenity. Herbalist Ellen Evert Hopman writes that a three-day tincture of the blossoms in vinegar makes a sort of holy water which is effective in dispelling unwanted energies from the home. The abundance and hardiness of the red clover renders it potent in a magical charm with protective or wealth-bringing intent. Children tend to be drawn to the red clover, so the dried blossoms are effective in spells requesting fertility. Many couples intent on having children who meet with difficulty tend to experience the added stress of self-blame and strong desire. A pouch of red clover blossoms can be worn by each couple to soothe the nerves, remind the partners of their inherent fertility and magically invite the presence of children into one's life.

ℰ RED CLOVER AND RICE

fresh red clover blossoms, picked in the morning dew
short grain brown rice
garlic
rice vinegar or an herbal vinegar

If you can, enlist the help of children in picking blossoms. I like to pick by following the trail of the bees, plucking blossoms they have just visited. Wash the rice, then dry roast it in a cast-iron pan, shaking the pan over the flame until the nutty aroma of the rice rises. Bring the rice to a boil in a covered pot, then lower the flame and let the rice cook for forty minutes.

As the rice is simmering, separate the green bottoms from the blossoms; set them aside for the compost pile as you finely chop the flowers. Mince several cloves of garlic as well. When the rice is done, let it cool, add the garlic, blossoms, and season all with vinegar. This dish creates a perfect combination of protein and carbohydrates which is sustaining and satisfying to the body, particularly for those who suffer from sugar swings or feel overwhelmed by sudden hunger and weakness.

ℰ RED CLOVER COUGH SYRUP

1 ounce of whole dried red clover blossoms
boiled water
honey

Make sure you can see the whole dried blossom. I've listed several resources in the resource section of the book which lists excellent sources for whole dried red clover blossoms. Be sure to order them around June, as the gathering season lasts only through mid-September.

Though most flower infusions only require ten minutes to two hours of infusing time, red clover blossoms sit for the full four hours, because the plant's mineral richness requires a lengthier time to seep into the water.

After the infusion has sat for four hours, take a pint of the infusion and decoct it, according to the directions for black birch soda in the March chapter. Add some clover honey and a bit of brandy and use this syrup when experiencing the type of cough that sounds like a car engine trying to turn over (this is known as a "dry, hacking cough").

While many of us easily experience the expansiveness of summer and joyfully move into the world of thinly clad bodies and late night celebration, at some point in our lives, most of us experience a summer where we feel oppressed by the heat, overwhelmed by crowds and longingly wish for a summer resort that looks like an igloo at the North Pole. As Janice Longboat aptly mentions, summer is hard on the heart, and for those whose hearts are heavy, summer is not welcomed but rather dreaded.

In my experience, I find that suppressing grief makes its pain keener. Comforting oneself when the heart is heavy can sometimes alleviate the heavy-chested feeling which accompanies grief or at least vent tears which need to flow. Herbal teas are also useful at this time, and many herbs which flower in the hot summer sun penetrate the cold, gray, and lifeless mists which surround and seem to cling to the grieving person. I find that lemon balm *(Melissa officionalis)* is exceptionally effective in brightening dim spirits. This herb, a traditional favorite for calming testy, "hyperactive" children, calms summer grumbling and truly lightens a heavy heart. Nicknamed melissa, lemon balm gladdens the spirits of those who become grim as Scrooge at Christmas as the hot sun turns their feet to lead and singes their eyelashes. Picked fresh, prepared as an infusion, and served iced like lemonade, lemon balm quenches thirst and clears the mind dampened by humidity. Lemon balm restores the gift of laughter to the grief-laden soul.

While there are times in our lives when we are struggling for our freedom, for the fulfillment of our hopes, dreams, and desires, July's natural abundance allows us to experience a sense of thriving and fullness through simple acts such as cooking, picking flowers, watching the garden vegetables ripen, and beholding the star-scattered sky. As the vegetables and grains come into readiness for food and storage, the summer moon sits glowing in yellow fullness just over the horizon's edge, sharing her fulsome beauty with all beings.

Perhaps because the shape of the full moon evokes wholeness, and its eerie silver light illuminates the darkness, the full-faced moon is considered in the realm of magic to be the phase in which we call our deepest desires into being, where we imagine and spin our thoughts and ideas into thriving reality. Whatever we wish to see come to fruition in our lives is offered to the light of the moon; the divine, magical power within the full moon blesses these desires with silver glow and the promise of fulfillment. I find my hidden, most treasured desires well up in response to the extravagant illumination and wild fullness of the moon.

If you are fortunate to live away from incessant, electrical outdoor lighting and near a woodland path, silently walking amidst trees under the light of the full moon keens our senses to the rustling excitement all creatures experience under the moon's orb. As the white beams of the moon enter our pores, our ancient, primal desire for freedom quickens, rises, and sends us roaming in search of long-suppressed wildness.

This month, find out the time of the full moon by consulting a lunar calendar or the *Farmer's Almanac.* Set aside an hour or two to sit and watch the moon. It is especially thrilling to view the moon with a small group of people who all give their attention to watching, and to have a special outdoor spot from which to observe the moon. In cities, one might go to the roof of one's building and view from there. A friend of mine has a star-watching rock in her backyard which she and her children sit upon for moon gazing. The tops of hills or small mounds which overlook flat farmland often give a spectacular view of the moon as she slowly reveals her full beauty to all on earth. The ocean acts as a glimmering mirror of the moon's light. If you are unable to devote this much time to moon gazing, watch the moon on and off throughout the full moon night. As the moon begins to rise, view her silent ascent with full awareness. When the moon appears just above the horizon, she often reveals her face with startling hugeness. Once the moon has climbed high in the sky, stand with firm legs and stretch your arms above your head, palms facing upward to draw the light of the fully risen moon down into the body. In European folk tradition, this stance was assumed in order to charge one's whole being with the rippling, wild power of the full moon. Inhale deeply, pulling the moonlight down to the soles of the feet. Keep the arms raised until you feel filled from head to toe with humming energy.

Then let your arms fall and gaze at the moon, naming your desire to thrive. Ask La Luna, in your own way, to keep the bloom in your cheeks, humor in your heart, to gift you with a robust body. Bare your soul to the moon, spilling before her the sacred truth of all that you want. The moon loves desire and will shine the light of her blessing onto your wishes. Give thanks to the moon for its constancy, its beauty and leave a wine glass full of water in the path of its beams all night long. Drink the water at once the following morning, or pour it into an opaque flask, sipping it through the month. Splash the roots of trees, the heads of flowers with the magic of moonwater, cooling the green nations as the summer air grows wiltingly hot, and then hotter still.

AUGUST

❧

Harvesting, Blessing

I CALL AUGUST the month of gold, for the fields that bestow upon us the earth's agricultural riches and for the slant of sun in the northeast United States, which casts a shimmering yellow light over all things. Gold too, is the full moon which rises so perfectly round and gilded, and the ripe corn which protects its rows of sweet yellow pouches in flaxen tassels of silk. Islands of intensely yellow goldenrod flowers undulate in the shifting winds, drawing spiders, ants, and bees with their sweet pollen; countryside farmstands and outdoor urban markets overflow with an abundance of vegetables, herbs, and fruit.

As we look deeply into the activities of the natural world in August, we see the energy of ripening and fruition take hands with the energy of death and decay; together they dance the dance which begins to bring autumn into being. Even as we bend low to pick squash and fill our baskets with tomatoes, calendula blossoms, and basil, even as we savor the blackberries whose ebony absorbs and reflects the sheen of the sun, summer begins to call back her dogged heat and the vivid brilliance of her flowers. Underneath the humid gusts of August wind, which bring a hissing song from the trees, lies the subtle, barely perceptible moulding leaf-scent of fall. The leaves of just a few plants begin to curl and wither, and the petals of many flowers drop to the ground as seed pods swell in preparation for the season of decay.

The unprobing eye, however, absorbs only the lushness and plenty in nature this month. As my own eyes survey the miracle of fruition, I am reminded of the European earth goddess Habondia, her braided hair thick as loaves of oven-baked bread, her arms pliant as dough yet supple and strong from outdoor labor, her long skirts colorful and well-pocketed to carry the bounty of the harvest and share it with all.

The ripening of the barley, the flowering of the goldenrod, and the readiness of the corn all come from the generous land embodied by this luxuriant goddess. The purpling of the plums and the reddening blush of the apple fruits mirror the healthful bloom in her cheeks and the swelling of the gourds matches the mounting ripeness of the goddess to womanhood. Habondia's lush physicality teaches us to be proud of abundance in all forms on earth, be it our own ample and curved flesh, the fruits of her joyous labor or the endless river of human imagination which brims its banks, flooding us with poetry, dance, song, story, meal-making, and ritual. She invites us to savor, celebrate, and create with the gifts of the land and to remember that we are worthy of these gifts.

Habondia's spirit is meant to remind us that abundance is our birthright, and that through the act of gathering to ourselves the harvest of nature we accept and relish this cycle of ripeness and fullness as well as our worthiness to receive treasure. Spilling her vast riches before us, Habondia challenges us to use our creativity to preserve some of the harvest, that it can sustain us through the long winter months. She asks only that we have gratitude for our full baskets and that we share what we have with others through the gift of our hospitality.

In the Celtic tradition, the first of August is marked by the festival Lughnasad, named after the sun god Lugh. Lugh's strength begins to wane at midsummer, when the daylight begins to decrease in length. As the sickle cuts through the first fully ripened sheaf of grain, the power of this god, known also as John Barleycorn, or the Green Man, leaps into the barley and the god dies. Lugh is called, thanked and honored through games, dances, and songs, both in gratitude for giving his life to preserve and nourish the cycle of life within the human community, and in the hopes of coaxing his fertile power, now embedded in the grain, to fullness as the harvest progresses.

The celebration of the harvest's beginning was accompanied by an understanding that the outcome of the harvest was unknown, that the still-growing crops were dependent on the amount of rain and that even in August a prolonged dry spell could cause the crops to wither. This fragility brought the people together, united in their intent to encourage growth and call upon the greater, unseen forces for assistance, for much work was still to be done to reap the bounty of the land.

HARVESTING

The very act of harvesting, of plucking fully formed vegetables and fruits from vines, stalks, and briars, kindles a sensuous connection to the miracle of growth and sustenance. My first summer in upstate New York, I went to a strawberry farm with some friends to pick a pint of this luscious fruit. I wore a wide-brimmed hat someone lent me and carried a woven willow basket in the hollow of my elbow. I began my walk to the far field while the sun was fading to orange and the glaring heat of the day softened into late afternoon shadow. As I entered the field, the cool, dark land welcomed my footsteps, adjusting her body to accommodate my weight. The gentle warmth of the air enveloped and seemed to accept me into what felt like a hospitable home. The wind coursed through my hair, jostling my hat; the feel of the basket sliding back and forth across my inner elbow as I strode toward the strawberries filled me with euphoric delight.

I reached the rows where some others bent, hats hiding their faces as they concentrated on their picking. I squatted down, my feet sinking into and becoming filmy with the grit of loosely turned earth, the warm sun at my back slowly dropping into the horizon. Basket beside me, I stretched out my arms, shifting my balance to catch hold of the reddest fruit. As I plucked each berry, I began to notice that the sweetest ones seemed to willingly give themselves to me, sliding into my fingers without any force on my part. The mound of seed-speckled, heart-shaped fruit grew taller, and the thought of sharing the contents of my basket with my housemates quickened my already throbbing heart. The deep joy and fulfillment I experienced in this first moment of direct exchange with the earth foreshadowed and ignited my heart's longing to know the plants deeply, and to learn to prepare food and medicine with them.

When we give ourselves to the act of harvesting, of separating leaves to expose the singular shape of a vegetable or fruit, when we pause and really see the extraordinary miracles growing to fullness before our eyes, we cannot help but be inspired by the ferocious originality of the creative force expressed in nature. Gathering food directly from the ground with our hands, dirt tracing the creases of skin in our palms and becoming embedded in our fingernails, gives birth to the desirous pulse within ourselves to create acts and articles of kindred beauty.

To me, work with the plants at harvest time is a gentle, powerful, and skillful tool for gradually repairing experiences of death, lack, and emptiness which were never followed by the subsequent energy of renewal, leaving instead a trail of distrust in the psyche. For food reaped by our own hands contains within it more than the sustenance of vitamins and minerals. With each bite we eat the entire experience of our gathering: the sun, the smell of the air, the temperature of that day, the people and beings we encountered in our gathering, and the sore but elated feel of our bodies which worked to harvest. We absorb the wild energy of food just weaned from the earth and an almost mysterious, unnameable nourishment fills our whole being, as the basket has been filled, with satisfaction.

For the herbalist, August is an industrious month. Plants which were gathered and left to steep in various mixtures from mid-May through June are ready to be decanted. As I stand at the kitchen counter and funnel preparations through cheesecloth to separate matrix from plant matter, my thoughts turn back to the hours spent gathering those plants, to the places I knelt in to gather, and to the students and friends who waded through field and forest with me in search of magic and medicine. My vision also leaps ahead toward fall and winter; I let my intuition guide me toward choosing the flowers, leaves, roots, barks, and berries I may need for my own health and for the well-being of my family and community. Though I do not harvest with sickle and scythe in large grainfields, I too look forward and plan what, when, and how to gather and keep the plants which will sustain myself and others until spring.

Season after season, year after year of gathering has slowly uprooted my linear-based conception of time and planted within me a more cyclical, spirallic sense of time's movement based on the rhythm of plants and trees in my own region. This newer, yet anciently familiar cycle has gifted me with a slowly burgeoning sense that I belong within the northeastern landscape. I await each month, familiar in its feel, seeking and marking the return of particular plants which bloom or cast seed at the same time each year. Still, the emergence of a particular flower within its anticipated month delights and surprises me like the unexpected visit of a dear friend.

In August the elements dance together in a way which readies the ground for a great medicine plant to come into full bloom. This plant's leaves and summer flowers assist us with the most stubborn of winter's illnesses, and the deepest of cuts, applying its shielding, reparative power magically as well as medicinally.

YARROW *(Achillea millefolium)*

Bone-white clusters of blooming yarrow interrupt the sheets of green and hay-colored grass that describe the fields and waysides of August, their striking presence pulling my wandering legs through meadows toward them. I pause to relish the spice and feel of this strong-stalked plant before harvesting it for its powerful medicine ways. Dozens of small, cream-white florets 'of yarrow crown its stick-straight stalk; the feathery gray-green leaves shimmer and bend in the hot breeze, adorning the grass with a silver cast.

While the finely cut leaf segments of yarrow appear soft and delicate, one tug on its soft leaves reveals the stubborn solidness of this plant: yarrow's ability to resist and remain grounded as one pulls the plant is a signature of its skill in resisting unbalancing forces. This strength gives yarrow the medicine to both resist and transform infection within the body, as well as its folkloric reknown as a plant offering psychic protection. This power of perseverance characterizes yarrow's healing style: its medicine permeates the deep layers of the body and settles to work in the subterranean pathways: arterial blood, the gastrointestinal tract, the womb and the bone marrow.

In western European, northern European, and Native American traditions yarrow is well known as a "vulnerary," that is, a wound-healing plant. Its Latin name, *Achillea millefolium*, refers to the warrior Achilles, who presumably used the plant successfully in stanching the wounds of his soldiers. One tale recounts that at his birth, Achilles' mother dipped him in a bath of yarrow tea, rendering him almost invulnerable. The heel by which she held the infant remained untouched by the brew, and it was into Achilles' yarrow-free heel the fatal arrow flew.

Yarrow's power as a wound healer has been unsurpassed for centuries, during which the plant has accumulated many folknames, such as nosebleed, woundwort, and carpenter's weed, all affectionate references to yarrow's fame as a wound herb. A snuff of the leaves was often used to effectively dam a copiously bleeding nose; the bitter oil kept the sinuses open and the antihemorrhage qualities halted the flow of blood. The snuff also assuaged the aching head.

The popular Chinese oracle, the *I Ching*, was originally cast using stalks of yarrow rather than coins. In eastern countries, the herb was called yarroway and was used in quite a unique manner to foretell one's romantic future. The inside of the nose was tickled with a serrated leaf as one spoke the following words: "Yarroway, yarroway, bear a white blow, If my love love me, my nose will bleed now." If the nose began to bleed, it was taken as an omen of love returned. One of yarrow's more infamous names was devil's plaything, a title probably given by the church, which discouraged the villager's use of plants for divination and spell work. Such practices were considered evil, and all evil fell under the dominion of the Christianity-created Devil.

Yarrow's leaves and flowers are antiseptic, antibacterial, styptic, anti-inflammatory, and astringent. These qualities combine to make yarrow my herb of choice to apply to both shallow and deep wounds. The antiseptic, antibacterial qualities of the plant prevent infection; its styptic ability stanches blood flow, its anti-inflammatory and astringent abilities reduce swelling. Yarrow leaves and flowers act as a potent anodyne, or pain-reliever, lightly numbing traumatized nerve endings. Due to its highly antibacterial nature, yarrow can be dried, powdered, and sprinkled directly on open wounds without the risk of causing infection.

Yarrow is even safe to apply externally to a cut which has opened the skin to the bone. The plant adeptly prevents infection and speeds tissue repair, quickly closing the wound without leaving any infection behind.

I have used yarrow extract on surface cuts as well, daubing it to sterilize wounds where wood or glass is embedded in the skin and needs to be extracted with tweezers. Spit poultices of yarrow deftly quench the pain and swelling of bee stings and shrivel blood blisters. The dried flowers steeped in boiled water and applied to the gums are incredibly effective for easing the pounding mouth pain which often follows dental work of any kind. When the novocaine begins to wear off, the yarrow offers similar relief, the poultice numbing the area directly underneath the plant matter while preventing the onset of infection in any open, gaping wounds in the mouth. A mouthwash of yarrow flowers and sage leaves reduces gingivitis and keeps the gums in healthy condition.

Warrior-like yarrow is specific for working with bruises from a violent origin. In New York City, a fellow garden member who played the fiddle was mugged the day he had scheduled an evening performance. When he showed me his swollen arm, I immediately directed him to the yarrow plant, where he chewed the leaves and applied them directly to his bruised bicep. Within minutes, the spit poultice numbed the pain and reduced the muscular swelling to a startling degree; the diaphoretic quality of yarrow opened his skin's pores and drew out the heat and infection. By late evening, he was able to carry on his performance as planned.

Yarrow is an excellent emergency care herb. A friend's ten-year-old daughter accidentally shut the car door on her bare foot as we were leaving for a day at the beach. Luckily, we were parked at the entrance to the garden; I rushed in, picked a handful of leaves, and thrust them into her mother's mouth, who chewed the leaves and covered her daughter's foot with the green mush. Within minutes the pain dissipated and we were able to take our ocean journey.

Yarrow's multifaceted healing gifts extend into the area of winter medicine. The late herbalist Adele Dawson reports that in the early eighteenth century, the Canadian Micmac Indians used the herb in sweat baths to relieve colds. Qualities of astringency, antibacterial *and* diaphoretic action in a plant often indicate usefulness in working with infectious colds and flus. Yarrow flowers open the pores of the skin and draw out fever; in traditional remedies it is combined with elder and peppermint in tea to promote a sweating fever which guides the flu out of the body.

As one strokes yarrow's silky leaves, the peppery, slightly bitter, sharply clear scent of its volatile oils is left on the hands. These volatile oils tighten inflamed tissues and open the nasal passageways, reducing pain and pressure and allowing air to flow more freely through the sinus cavity. I have had tremendous success with yarrow in the realm of sinus infections, sipping the hot flower tea, or taking a dropperful of extract three times a day when acute sinus pain or bleeding is present. Yarrow offers comfort and relief on the first day of a cold, quickly drying up runny noses and moving fever, its sweat-promoting capacity hastening the healing process.

Yarrow is a powerful herb for women, working skillfully to alter and relieve a multitude of woman-specific challenges. Yarrow's astringent and hemostatic abilities have called herbalists to use the plant as a poultice, salve, and tea when working with hemorrhoids and varicose veins, conditions which often accompany pregnancy and childbirth. Combined with shepherd's purse during labor, yarrow prevents uterine hemorrhage. Midwives apply poultices of the leaves to nipples which are sore and infected from breastfeeding, and recommend sitz baths of the plant to repair perineal tears. Drunk several days before the menses are due, yarrow can slow profuse menstrual flow, and is sometimes effective in checking menopausal flooding.

Yarrow eases the sense of inner restlessness which sometimes arises during the menopausal years and, according to herbalist Kate Gilday, is a specific ally for women who felt strong in youth but experience a loss of that sturdiness as they go through menopause. The plant's diaphoretic quality may increase the sweating that accompanies hot flashes, so care must be taken when choosing this herb to decrease menstrual flooding. Yarrow promotes the production of progesterone, a hormone helpful in slowing the too-frequent menstrual cycles which can occur in the early menopausal years. Yarrow can also be used to promote rhythmic menstrual flow in young women and is a specific ally for women who feel clumsy the week before they bleed. As with all amphoteric herbs, the plant seems to intuitively assess which action is needed to restore internal balance.

Taken as a tea, yarrow slowly and steadily works to shrink fibroids. Prepared as a sitz bath it is effective in checking the bleeding that accompanies these common, sometimes painful tumors. The volatile oils in yarrow, which are most potent in plants that have been gathered in the midday sun, work to break up blood congestion in the pelvic area; practitioners of traditional Chinese medicine name "stagnant" blood as the cause of amenorrhea, fibroids, and dysmenorrhea. Yarrow applies her persistence in the womb to gradually transform these conditions. The plant's hemostatic quality relieves bleeding in the lungs and stomach as well as the womb.

Yarrow sitz baths are a favorite healing tool of Swiss herbalist Maria Treben, who states simply that "women could be spared many troubles, if they just took yarrow tea from time to time." Maria holds that yarrow regulates the bodily juices, and stimulates the production of fresh blood cells in the bone marrow. The tannins in yarrow, imparted to the bathwater, give the plant an astringency which revivifies prolapsed uterus, relieves vaginal itching, and dries excessive vaginal mucus. The bath used to relieve itching should be followed by a cup of warm tea and a period of twenty minutes sweating under the bedcovers.

In Austria, yarrow is known as *Bauchwehkrautl*, the bellyache herb. Sheep and goats seek out and munch the plant when they are in digestive distress. The plant's bitter taste is a signpost of its skill with gastrointestinal disorders. Acting on the mucus membranes, yarrow eases indigestion and heartburn, disperses the intestinal heat which accompanies colitis, and checks inflammation of the diverticula in the intestinal tract. Yarrow tea and tincture relieve gas and ease headaches caused by liver distress. Sipped hot, yarrow regulates bowel movements and eases pressure and heaviness in the stomach region. Yarrow effectively halts abdominal cramping.

The antibacterial and astringent qualities of yarrow work to disinfect the urinary tract, reducing infection in and toning the bladder. Yarrow relieves incontinence and heals interstitial cystitis, a condition where noninfectious ulcerations appear in the bladder wall. Old herbals recommend the tea as a wash through the scalp to check hair loss; this action is possibly due to the plant's rich thiamine content, a vitamin which calms the nervous system. A salve of the flowers also works well for this purpose and is particularly useful when working with hair loss resulting from radiation, chemotherapy, and hormonal imbalance. The plant can be carried, inhaled, and ingested to neutralize the effects of radiation. Siberian ginseng and miso can also be taken during this time to prevent damage from radiation.

The flower essence of yarrow gives psychic protection against draining energies and my own sense is that as the bitter, volatile principles of the plant clear the sinus passageways, respiration deepens as well as one's ability to clearly "sniff out" situations for the purpose of self-protection. The lore around yarrow lauds its prowess in offering the bearer magical protection. The plant is believed to grow where the earth's ley lines are strong, guarding those areas and calling the attention of those who recognize this silent indication of sacred space. Sitting in locales of yarrow revivifies one's own energy field.

An herb of Venus, one old spell uses yarrow, sewn up in a flannel and placed under the pillow, to bring visions of one's future husband or wife. The following words were repeated: "Thou pretty herb of Venus tree, Thy true name is yarrow; Now who my bosom friend must be, Pray thou tell me tomorrow."

In North America, wild yarrow flowers are usually ivory colored, while in Europe the flowers are often light to deep pink. In Switzerland, the pink variety is considered the most potent for medicinal use, and here the white flowers are coveted. When making preparations from yarrow, I use only flowers and leaves I have gathered in the wild, and here, on the east coast, the cream-colored flowers are the most abundant. Yarrow's creamy petals and yellow centers remind me of the union of the August sun and moon; I love to preserve their finely divided, toothy shaped leaves and orange-flecked, pearly corymbs by pressing them between the pages of a thick book.

☙ YARROW FLOWER ESSENCE

a sunny, dry morning
untreated spring water
fresh yarrow flowers
brandy
a glass bowl
amber bottles
labels
a dropper bottle

On a sunny day, in the late morning, find an area where the yarrow flowers are growing in abundance. Sit quietly with the flowers for a while, resting the mind and body. Filling a bowl with water, pick the blossoms, and float them on the surface of the water in the bowl. It is best to pluck the flowers from just down the stem, to avoid touching the petals. Pick enough flowers to cover the surface of the water with petals. Place the bowl in bright sunlight for three hours. (If the blossoms begin to fade, do not wait the three hours.) After three hours, remove the blossoms by hand from the bowl, touching the water as little as possible. Fill the amber bottles half way with the spring water, and add an equal amount of brandy per bottle as a natural preservative. This liquid forms the mother essence. Dosage bottles are prepared by adding two drops of mother essence into a one-ounce dropper bottle of water, with several drops of brandy to preserve the water. With each dilution, lightly tapping or shaking the bottle releases the energy of the essence. This preparation is effectively used when one must be around unpleasant human influence.

☙ YARROW FLOWER OIL

yarrow blossoms and leaves
olive oil
jar

Follow the instructions for making oils in the March chapter. This oil is wonderful for the scalp, on skin which is about to be or has been exposed to radiation, and can be made into a salve with the usual addition of beeswax for frequent application to wounds.

℮ YARROW SITZ BATH

2 cups of yarrow blossoms/whole yarrow herb (if possible)
cold or boiled water
a jar

Sitz baths are taken with the tub filled only to the level of the kidneys; the whole body is not immersed. Leaving the upper body free is important because certain herbs quicken the circulation; often, while we want to increase limb circulation, we do not want to increase the pumping of blood around the heart area. Sitz baths are used in general for healing involving the anal and genital area as well as the kidneys. There are several ways to prepare the infusion for sitz baths. One way is to make a standard infusion (see directions in the March chapter) and add to hot bathwater. Maria Treben recommends steeping a generous amount of whole yarrow in cold water overnight, boiling the brew in the morning, and adding to the bath.

Yarrow's diaphoretic action, magnified in steaming water, makes the sitz bath useful for drawing out fever. In addition to its work with fibroids mentioned above, yarrow sitz baths also prevent infection and speed healing of perineal tears. Some women find yarrow baths so astringent they feel a bit dried out in the perineal area. I recommend annointing the labia with an emollient herbal oil or salve such as violet or chickweed (avoid if you have an open wound) after you emerge from the bath.

e↝   YARROW FOMENTATION

yarrow leaves and flowers, fresh or dried
boiled water
a washcloth

Pour boiled water over the herbs and let the brew steep for ten minutes. When the brew has cooled to body temperature or a bit hotter, dip the cloth into the tea and apply it to cuts and blisters. This method is particularly effective for speedy healing of the blistering sores which accompany impetigo.

e↝   YARROW MOUTHWASH

yarrow flowers
sage leaves
plantain leaves
boiled water
a touch of brandy or vinegar
quart jar

The combined disinfectant, antibacterial and astringent qualities of these herbs make a fine wash for the teeth and gums. Prepare a standard infusion of the herbs, discard the leaf matter and add several ounces of vinegar or brandy to the brew. Refrigerate. Another way to work with the mouthwash is to prepare a standard tincture from fresh yarrow, sage, and plantain (*Plantago major*) leaves, separately, and add a dropperful of each tincture to a cup of water before rinsing one's mouth.

As I began to bring the section on yarrow to a close, another plant nudged at my side, reminding me of a wintertime promise I had made to share its gifts here. A close friend of the sun, this famous herb carries summer warmth in its hardy leaves throughout the year, offering us heat and many other magical and medicinal gifts in a simple cup of tea.

ROSEMARY *(Rosmarinus officinalis)*

Until just this summer, when I called rosemary to mind, I saw fragrant wreaths and small, potted herbs sitting on the kitchen windowsill within easy reach of both my hands and the sun's rays. Then I remembered one particularly large rosemary shrub which sat in the window of a twelfth-floor office I worked in many years ago. The mission of this organization was to preserve and disseminate the teachings of an anthroposophic philosopher, and the office space was unique in that a room was set aside for meditation. Twice a day, most of the employees quietly disappeared into a small room to visualize world peace.

Whether or not they were directly successful, the plants in the office were remarkably vital, and the rosemary shrub in particular grew deep green and thick-barked. The office accountant, a Czechoslovakian woman, decided to retire, and as we stood by the coffee machine one day, she asked me if I knew anyone who would want to take the rosemary plant. For reasons left unexplained, she could not keep the plant herself but was loathe to leave it behind. When she heard I had a garden, her eyes widened and she insisted that I take the rosemary. She said she would rest easy knowing the plant she had watered for eight years would finally feel fresh air on its leaf tips.

I hesitated. My own gardening experience was limited to cultivating weeds, wild plants which required little prodding. I mumbled that the soil's lead count in our garden was questionable and, well . . . I left the office with my arms wrapped around a huge clay pot, the rosemary trembling with each of my footsteps. The plant was so large I had to peer through its leaves to see my way home.

Several curious things happened as I walked east, heading toward my garden. The scent of the plant grew more and more pungent, and people began to stop me, leaning over to smell the leaves and affectionately stroking the plant. Some folk smiled mutely and moved on, and others spoke a sentence or two, absently fingering the plant as they referred dreamily to their mother's cooking, their grandmother's garden, or of a Mediterranean location where they'd met the apparently unforgettable rosemary. By the time I turned down First Avenue, the location of several long-standing Italian homemade pasta and cheese shops and the home of the matriarch-run Sicilian pizzeria, the elderly relatives of these storekeepers nodded firmly not at me, but at rosemary.

The more attention rosemary got, the stronger she put out her unmistakable perfume. I watched people pause in conversation and sniff the air as the smell of the plant wafted toward them, overpowering bus fumes, defying car exhaust, and shocking nonplussed New Yorkers to attention. People actually turned their heads as I walked by. I found myself standing taller, as if my beloved and I were walking down the street hooked arm in arm. I began to feel regal, utterly awake and clear, abandoning the usual shielding habits I applied while walking through Manhattan's streets.

Liberated from its twelfth-floor office window, released from its climate-controlled environment and loosed upon the real world, the rosemary shrub was, without a doubt to my mind, singing a freedom song with her smell. This extraordinary encounter with rosemary was the first time I experienced a plant as a responsive being. By the time I relieved my arms of the heavy planter and laid it gently in my garden, I was merry and drunk with love. Rosemary, however, was clearly *not* monogamous.

The lore of rosemary is as vast as the Mediterranean Sea upon whose sandy shores the plant's bare roots cling. All who come into contact with the herb are blessed with the gift of remembrance. The most well-known reference to rosemary comes from Shakespeare's *Hamlet*, where Ophelia in her madness, casts a sprig onto the ground saying: "There's rosemary for you, that's for remembrance! Pray you love, remember." A superb tonic for the memory, rosemary tones the mental faculties of those of all ages, but of elders in particular, keeping their memories intact.

Rosemary is a special ally for elderly storytellers, aiding them in accurately preserving and telling the stories which keep us linked to our heritage and help us understand the weathers that have shaped our families. Rosemary's skill with enhancing memory has made the herb a prime magical choice for the lover who wishes to inspire fidelity in his or her partner. Brides often wear twined wreaths of rosemary, and the plant is presented to wedding guests as a symbol of friendship.

The wild folk and peasants held that rosemary would only grow well in a house where women were the dominating force. The belief was so widespread that many kitchen gardens sported crippled rosemary plants which had been injured by the men of the household in the hopes of destroying evidence of their inferior authority. Rosemary was also revered by the Spaniards as one of the bushes that gave shelter to the Virgin Mary. Imagining the rosemary plants I'd seen in our local farmer's market, it seemed that the Virgin Mother would have had to crouch rather low or performed a miracle herself to hide underneath a rosemary bush.

However, when I visited France, I came across dense hedgerows of rosemary which served to shield houses that would otherwise have been in full view of the road. As I wandered through the gardens of a castle in Dover I came across luxuriant, long-haired vines of rosemary draped over the tiers that formed the estate garden's terraced borders. Mary would clearly have found shelter beneath these rosemarys.

Amongst the Sicilians is a belief that young fairies take the form of snakes and lie among rosemary's pungent branches. In Italy and Spain the plant is considered a safeguard against witches; this familiar phrase often indicates that the village wise women—later called witches—used the plant frequently and with success. Much like lavender, rosemary was burned with juniper berries to purify the air and prevent infection. An old French name for the herb was *incensier*, for it was burned in churches as an inexpensive incense.

Rosemary is astringent, stomach-healing, stimulant, and antispasmodic. Its primary effects are felt in the head, the stomach, and the heart. Rosemary relieves headaches, and a sprig or two taken as a simple tea or eaten in salads daily will slowly improve memory and increase mental acuity. The volatile oil in the leaves stimulates a sluggish liver and relieves headaches which are the result of digestive torpor. The vapors of steamed rosemary purify the air, and inhaling the steam dispels depression, lifts the spirits, and increases one's zest for life. Herdsmen in the east encouraged their flocks to feast on rosemary for the pleasing taste it imparted to the milk.

Early herbals recommend the plant for those who are feeble, suffer from sourness, or have lost their appetite. Rosemary's diuretic quality relieves edema and puffiness in old folks' feet. The leaves boiled in white wine and rinsed over the face were said to keep the face "faire"; taken internally, the same brew eased coughs. The gypsies of the Mediterranean peddled a toilet water called "Queen of Hungary's water," after Elizabeth, the Queen of Hungary in 1235, used a preparation of distilled rosemary flowers as a rinse to keep her face youthful-looking. The gently astringent property of the plant tightens the pores and the volatile oils bring circulation to the face. This water was splashed on the faces of those who fainted, effectively reviving them, and confirming rosemary's virtue as a nervine.

Queen of Hungary's water was also said to swiftly cure headaches and can be found for sale today in older parts of cities in both Europe and Central America. Employing rosemary's antiseptic quality, the gypsies applied a powdered form of the leaves to the umbilical cords of newborn infants and kept small pillows stuffed with leaves under the heads of sleeping children to prevent nightmares. Wandering gypsy bands hung wreaths of rosemary in the doorways of their caravans to protect against evil forces.

According to Juliette Levy, the gypsies revered rosemary for its effect on the blood; they used the plant as a heart tonic, for checking high blood pressure, for preventing miscarriage, and in cases of "impure" blood. As the liver is the primary organ which filters the blood, the gypsies were "cleansing" the bloodstream by calling upon rosemary's liver-stimulating skill. Sun-loving, strong-smelling rosemary is an invigorating plant: the herb's volatile oils and tannins stimulate blood, awaken the brain, promote appetite, and dispel sluggishness in both body and spirit.

An old herbal recommends burning the wood of rosemary, baking bread on this fire, and feeding the bread to those suffering from asthma or emphysema. The dried leaves can also be smoked as tobacco to dispel coughs and bronchial conditions. As a stomachic, rosemary was said to quiet the stomach and keep the breath fresh by promoting healthy digestion. I believe rosemary's nervine property calms digestion disturbed by anxiety and worry.

Today, one of rosemary's most well-known uses is as a hair tonic. The infused oil is superb for preventing unnatural falling of hair, and can successfully protect the scalp and hair when one is undergoing radiation or chemotherapy. The oils in rosemary stimulate follicle growth, brighten the hair, and prevent baldness. A powerful insecticide, rosemary tea can be applied to the skin to repel mosquitoes, mayflies, and deer-flies. Rosemary extends her protectiveness to neighboring plants and orchards, where the herb's scent repulses insects. Externally, rosemary can be applied to bites and stings.

Rosemary's Latin name, *Rosmarinus*, means "dew of the sea," a reference to the ocean spray which forms beads of water on the shrub's leathery leaves and gives the plant a magical sheen. For those who desire everlasting youth, gather the morning dew off of rosemary or lady's mantle leaves, cupping your hand under the leaf and bending the plant so the dew flows into your palm. Cover your face in this cool liquid which is the juice of dawn.

I eventually brought that large rosemary plant to my father's garden in Brooklyn. A tender perennial, we decided Dad would keep rosemary indoors for the winter. By December the shrub grew so large I made several holiday wreaths of rosemary and rosehips as winter gifts. One day in February, my father called to tell me the rosemary plant, which he had taken to calling "she," had suddenly died. Neither of us could explain her dramatic turn for the worse and quick death. Many years later, while on a walk by the Hudson River just outside of the city, I ran into my old boss from that spiritual organization. She told me that the woman who gave me the rosemary had died of cancer the winter after she retired. The image of rosemary dropping all her leaves at once sprang immediately to mind; understanding the kinship which existed between the Czech woman and rosemary, I realized why the plant had died so abruptly.

While rosemary tea brings deep warmth to the body, the plant is a sensitive perennial and prefers to be taken indoors when the weather dips below freezing. I keep the plant in my kitchen in the winter, taking care to keep its roots connected to the soil it grew in while outdoors.

☙ ROSEMARY OIL

jojoba oil or a cold-pressed organic olive oil
fresh or dried rosemary leaves

Rosemary leaves are one of the few plants that can be infused in oil or
vodka fresh or dried. This is due to the leatheriness of the leaves, which
protect the volatile oils of the plant until they are released into a liquid
matrix. When making an infused oil from dried leaves, fill your jar only
one-third of the way, as the leaves will draw the olive oil into themselves
as they impart their own volatile oils to the matrix.

Rosemary infused in a fine olive oil is excellent for cooking. Steeped
in jojoba oil, it is fine hair tonic. When applying rosemary oil to help
hair growth, massage the oil *into the scalp* rather than on the hair. I find
that rosemary oil on my hair actually dries it out.

You may also want to experiment with preparing a rosemary oil, a
yarrow flower oil, and mixing the two and rubbing into the scalp, particularly if one is undergoing radiation or chemotherapy.

☙ ROSEMARY POTATOES

1 pound small round potatoes with yellow or red skins
½ cup rosemary oil
½ cup olive oil
fresh or dried rosemary leaves
garlic
a glass oven-safe bowl with a lid

Pour an equal amount of rosemary infused oil and olive oil into the bottom of the glass bowl and add the potatoes. Using both your hands, coat
the potatoes completely with the oil. Add the fresh or dried rosemary
leaves. I like to put these in whole; if the leaves are fresh, I bruise them a
bit to release their scent; if they are dry, I place the spindly leaves between my palms and then rub my hands against one another as if warm-

ing them, letting the slightly-crushed herbs fall into the bowl of potatoes. I like the dish to look generously scattered with rosemary's snaky-looking green leaves. Chop three or four cloves of garlic and sprinkle over the potatoes.

Place the prepared bowl, covered, in a 450° oven for about an hour. After about forty-five minutes, begin checking the potatoes for tenderness. You can also keep basting the potatoes in their oil every fifteen minutes or so during the entire cooking time. When the potatoes are almost tender, take the lid off and let the tops of the potatoes brown until slightly crispy.

Before serving you may want to add a bit more fresh garlic and rosemary. You won't easily forget this satisfying dish.

ROSEMARY MOTH REPELLENT

1 part dried rosemary leaves
2 parts dried wormwood leaves
1 part lavender flowers
a cloth and ribbon

When I use the word "parts" I am speaking of ratios. The total recipe is composed of four parts; wormwood comprises one-half of the final concoction, and each other herb, one-quarter. I like the idea of repellents because they allow the unwanted insects to withdraw, rather than killing them.

The cloth should be wide enough to fit the herbs in. Crush the leaves and flowers as you put them into the cloth, and then tie the bundle tightly with ribbon. You may want to baste the ribbon through the cloth, with a knot at one end, so the bag closes tightly. Keep the sachets in your drawers.

If you are using the mixture for clothes you are storing in chests or trunks for the summer, place an open cloth atop the clothes and sprinkled the dried leaves themselves on the cloth.

BLESSING

While a rich harvest may be our birthright, and we are truly children of the earth in that the earth mother is the provider of our food, shelter, and clothing, we only feel our affluence if we recognize the precious richness of these gifts by nurturing the rain, sun, and wind with our thanksgiving.

In Judaism thanksgiving is offered through the utterance of blessings: there is a blessing to be recited for each of life's commonplace activities. Taking a moment to give thanks for the blessing of a glass of water or wine, a hawk in flight, a slice of hot bread, renders these substances and events sacred. Moreover, the practice helps us become aware, through the habitual acts of our lives, that in truth we are the recipients of blessings many times each day. Blessings are a way we harvest the field of plenty which always surrounds us.

When the ancient, agriculturally bound rituals became absorbed into increasingly Christianized cultures, August's festival of the sun god, Lughnasad, was renamed Lammas, or Loaf Mass, by the Saxons. The god's reincarnation as the ripened grain was symbolized by two loaves of bread baked from the first-cut, husked, winnowed, and milled grain of the harvest season. One loaf was left at a crossroads in gratitude to the grain god and goddess; the other was distributed to the community, where it was blessed by all and eaten to represent the comingling of the human body with the fertile spirit of an earthy, green god. By eating the bread, one took in the spark of the god's vital force. This ritual has been absorbed into the Christian rite of communion.

This month, by the first eve of August (Lammas Eve) or before the moon waxes to full, locate a bakery where you can purchase several loaves of freshly baked, whole-grain bread, thickly crusted and studded with nuts or raisins. Choose loaves that remind your imagination of the roundness and fertility of Habondia and Lugh. If you feel greatly inspired, you can bake your own bread—kneading dough, sniffing its yeasty scent does much to help the desire to give blessing rise to the surface of one's consciousness.

When your loaves are ready, set up a small table or cloth at a crossroads, where spirits tend to flock, and leave a loaf out for them, in hopes of a fulfilling harvest. Bit by bit, tear off pieces of the second loaf, holding each portion up to the sun and saying a blessing for something in your life which brings you nutrition. For example, you can say: "Blessed is my dog Maura, for her loyalty and devotion sustain me." Or, "I bless my garden, for the opportunity it gives me to keep myself earthy and grounded." After you recite each blessing, eat the bit of bread.

Performing this simple ritual with a group of people can be quite uplifting. Each person has her own small loaf of bread, or a slice of a large loaf, and gives one blessing until the whole circle has had a chance to speak. Each person continues offering a blessing, going around and around the circle until the bread is gone.

All of August, continue to celebrate the blessings of creation springing out of the earth, sharing meals with friends and family, savoring ocean and lake, forest and meadow, before fall causes the warmth of the sun to recede. Each time you eye a loaf of bread, think back to the blessings you named, letting the memory of them bring you the sensation of fullness akin to that of the earth's fruition as you held them to you all month long. With the knowledge of the harvest strong in your bones, listen to the whisper of the leaves beginning to shiver on the branch as the slightly cooler night wind passes through them, bringing the first intimation of change to summer's landscape.

SEPTEMBER

c

Turning, Returning

IN SEPTEMBER THE countenance of the earth begins to turn again. The sylvan terrain through which the maiden rambled in spring, the sweeping fields and ripening gardens of high summer that grazed the mother's thighs as she gathered the gifts of the land, transform into yet another landscape. As the harvest deepens, the fullness of the mother within each plant stretches and fattens the fruits, vegetables, and grains to new limits of roundness. As the sun weakens, the life force divides, one fork beginning a slow journey back down the stalks of the plants toward the roots, and another maturing the seeds of all plants. The honeyed, yellow umbels of fennel flowers thicken into stomach-soothing crescents; the nodding ivory crowns of Queen Anne's lace turn their nestlike cups toward the ground, wild carrot seeds jostled and scattered by the first cool gusts of the coming autumn.

The whistling swell of the wind through the thinning spines and leaves of the plants reaches the ears of the crone, the ancient, aged wise woman who rises up from her underground lair and begins to walk the fields herself. She is the dark cloak that begins to wrap the earth as the hours of daylight wane. She both utters and is the piercing cry of the geese who gather and fly south. Goddess of decay, death, and rebirth, the crone summons the colors to the leaves and the cold to the land; it is she who gives the signal for the withering to begin and for all creatures to ready their homes for winter. Her knuckles the gnarled burls of tree trunks, the crone dresses the land in brown and touches all who live upon the earth with the desire to draw inward.

Hooded in the sable of the night sky, the crone advances, her footfall unhurried and deliberate upon the leaf-speckled soil. In a voice husky with woodsmoke, she summons home the abundant mother who is her daughter. And like most daughters, the mother sets loose a great surge of energy as her leave-taking draws near, unleashing a final ripeness which courses through all life. Gardens yield second harvests of basil, tomatoes, and lettuce, as butternut, acorn, and sweet dumpling squash gift us with their mouthwatering flesh and mineral-rich seeds. As the heat ebbs, summer drowsiness is replaced by a coolness which stirs our blood and invites us to enter a new cycle in which we gather, prepare and preserve both food and our own energy as the time of retreat draws near.

The provident earth-as-mother offers opulent fare at this time which ripens beneath the ground or close upon it, giving us hardy roots, tubers, and vegetables replete with starches, carbohydrates, and complex sugars. The chemistry of these foods lavish us with long-lasting, deeply satisfying nutrition our bodies can store and draw upon throughout the winter. Colorful, shapely, and uniquely textured, the magnificent and sensual booty of the fall harvest overflows the horn of plenty; nature's skillful marriage of utility and beauty inspires us to mirror this creative finesse as we cook foods and artfully craft symbols and rituals which carry us through the seasonal transition with joy and health. Even as we celebrate the magnificence of the abundant harvest, the subtle death-touch of the crone upon nature gently prods us to prepare for the season of introspection and contemplation, as winter will soon be upon us.

As a child, I remember another form of the Crone's call, a sound that spanned centuries and seas of culture; a cry that awakened a bird in my heart, a bird that stretched its wings, fluttered, and flew to promontories where rapt, uninterrupted listening brought communion with forces larger than myself. The call came from a spiralling ram's horn known as the shofar, blown in long and staccatoed blasts during the month of September by a rabbi in the Jewish synagogue. Akin to a magical incantation, the trumpeting cry of the shofar announced the beginning of the

Days of Awe. Its voice opened a window through which the past, present, and future poured, creating a loophole in time during which the inscription of a sorrowful destiny could be altered by celebration, devout prayer, fasting, and authentic remorse for one's regrettable actions.

What captured my young, life-seeking spirit was the hush that fell over the throng of murmuring worshipers as the rabbi unwrapped the twisted horn from its white silk shawl. His cheeks strained and reddened as he struggled to unleash the voice within the shofar. Even the strangled noises which first emerged from the coiled horn were a language that leapt beyond the sounds I experienced in the everyday din of the forgetful mechanical world. The shofar was a tether that spiraled back to preverbal history; its rasp wordlessly and instinctively linked me to a time where the sheer pulse of life was invoked and celebrated under the star-thick sky.

In the call of the shofar I saw sandals and bare feet strike the ground as if it were a drum; I smelled red earth, blood, and outdoor air sweetened by flowers and sharpened to clearness by the salt of the sea. I saw deer pause in their ground-nuzzling, bodies stone-still as they cocked their own horns toward the wailing speech. The shofar stirred an ocean of wildness which I didn't know, until that moment, lived in my memory, an ocean whose waves dove and crested with the pattern of the horn's cry.

The entire month of September follows a similar sinuous rhythm as the air wavers between heat and coolness and the landscape echoes the fullness and decay of the mother and crone. The color and density of the grasses shift in the face of these fluctuations, and the pitch of the wind's whistle alters into a stronger keen as it sweeps through the thinning skins of the leaves. The scent of molding leaves and weakening green life suffuse the air.

The turn of the season can be felt strongly at the autumnal equinox, when the hours of daylight and nightlight coincide, the dark beginning to override the light. The equinox offers us a pause where we can sense the moment of balance between light and dark through the internal mirror of our bodies and welcome the onset of this season where night reigns. To invite in the descent and darkness which begin at equinox ascribes to the dark a holiness which has become rare in this age of artificial, ever-available light. The time between harvest and spring becomes deeply devotional, internal, and mysterious rather than inconvenient and unproductive. Though it limits the breadth of our activity, the dark expands our ability to heal through rest, and to communicate with the world that speaks in the silence of night. The dark teaches us to seek and tend another fire, one that burns within us as the outer world dims.

Like a fisherman drawing in the nets he has dipped in the ocean, September's equinox quietly pulls in the light which filled each long day of summer. The chilling dusk signals all animals to hasten homeward, returning to the shore of our beings and preparing to take shelter within ourselves. The cooler September air brings a clarity and energy which assists us in readying for the impending winter. These transitional weeks between the seasons often create a window of vulnerability in our immunity through which illness enters. Our green allies can be called upon during summer's metamorphosis to bring us a constitutional hardiness and nourish the strength of organs and body systems most weakened by the cold.

The shifting, unpredictable atmosphere formed as each season tumbles to the next is a useful time to watch one's self deeply, to learn one's own habit patterns of waxing and waning energy. Understanding the bedrock limitations and strengths of our bodies allows us to more wisely choose a green ally which cradles our fragile underbelly, and, when possible, optimally transforms our health. The plant I have chosen for September may be controversial to those who are personally unfamiliar with its healing ways. However, my experiences with this herb have found it to be deeply loyal and indomitable, providing just the right combination of soothing and strengthening needed as the season changes and the cold arrives.

COMFREY *(Symphytum officinale)*

It would be impossible to even begin discussing comfrey without addressing the recent cautions and allegations made against it by the scientific community. But before I review the details of the laboratory tests upon which these findings were based, I must first draw you the profile of what I see when I am with the comfrey plant. I see strength. Tree trunk strength. I see rootedness, sturdiness, and flexibility employed in their right and proper times and places. I see irrepressible instinct for growth and regeneration. I smell the green wetness of nature which restores and awakens.

One spring, in Vermont, I attended a day-long herbal symposium, where I had the great pleasure of meeting herbalist Adele Dawson. Adele's frame was elfin; but at 86 she walked solidly, with the grace of a much taller woman, her posture erect and regal. Her mind was extraordinarily sharp, her humor intact. Accustomed to seeing most women of her age walk with the aid of a cane, I was struck by her surefootedness. I sat at her feet as she spoke about the herbs in her garden, winking her sparkling eyes as she offered tantalizing recipes for cordials using various garden favorites. I was tickled and struck at how often she was moved by *pleasure* to create tasty and medicinal herbal concoctions. When she began to discuss comfrey, she spoke as if referring to her closest friend, and firmly stated that she attributed her good health to drinking a single cup of comfrey leaf tea each day for thirty years.

Another impression of comfrey: I am at a yoga ashram for the month of September to earn a teaching certificate. We are being housed in draughty buildings devoid of any heat, the air laden with stagnant, heavy moisture. As we grow sicker each day, the swami of the ashram insists that we are cleansing: that our sniffles, sneezing, and coughs are irrefutable proof of our toxicity from living in New York City. However, the mint I have gathered and hung in my window will not dry, because the building's dampness is so great. I find the swami's attitude toward my body's natural response to this moldy, wet environment inhuman. I am shocked by the nodding heads, by those who accept his shaming assumptions; at a ritual in his trailer one evening, I notice the wood stove which keeps his quarters warmly livable. In this circumstance I am powerless over those whose self-trust and self-connection to their bodies has been hindered by the assumption that health means never getting sick, thwarting aging, and attempting to bypass death.

To assuage my anger, I flee daily to the garden, burying my hands in the earth to cool my rage, concentrating my love on that which I can trust and count on, the thick crowns and descending roots of comfrey, poke, and yellow dock. The ashram gardener—whom I have never seen at meditation—is an older man in overalls with sturdy arms and skin ruddy as red oak leaves. Seeing my joy at the profusion of comfrey, he offers me as much root as I like. He says that each year, while turning the soil, his spade inevitably breaks the comfrey roots, accomplishing a division which propagates dozens of baby comfrey plants come spring.

I hold the root to my nose as he speaks. Its smell is intoxicatingly earthy. When he talks about the curve of his spade splitting the comfrey and the plant's regeneration, I think of nature's ever-returning desire for life. The root I clutch in my hands is broad and black, its inner flesh white and so sticky my fingers are quickly and stubbornly webbed together by the gluelike, clear mucilage flowing from each nick in the root. Breaking off a piece and brushing off dirt, I pop a rootlet into my mouth, where it slips and slides, soothing my throat as I swallow it down. My stomach warms and unclenches. The gardener offers me chunks of the root, which I replant in small pots to bring home to my city garden.

The autumn wind and the rust colored, reliable mounds of the surrounding Catskill range clear all wisps of confusion from my mind. As I scoop palmfuls of earth into clay pots, I assure myself of what I am made of and conclude that it is not toxic. As the monthlong training progresses, I continue my daily work in the garden, the hairy, large leafed comfrey keeping me closely knit to my own truth about health, a truth that makes room for human strength and vulnerability and carries the gentle knowing of the plants within it. I hang peppermint, comfrey, and flowering yarrow leaves in the window of my dorm room. They mold and wither. Are these stalks "releasing toxicity," these plants which have known only rural life? No, they are simply responding to their conditions. And comfrey tea, demulcent, protein-rich, stomach-healing and bone-repairing, holds flu at bay, warming my damp toes and keeping the green of life running through my veins all month long.

In the 1970's, experimental data from Australia indicated that laboratory rats which had been fed comfrey showed liver damage due to pyrrolizidine alkaloids. The rats were fed several times their body weight of comfrey leaves over a long period of time. Another scientist in Japan reported that pyrrolizidine, potentially toxic to the liver and carcinogenic, existed in comfrey leaves. Herbalist Rosemary Gladstar, in her fine discussion of the comfrey controversy in *Herbal Healing for Women*, points out that pyrrolizidine, the alkaloid in comfrey which carries cell-inhibiting action, is balanced in the plant by cell builders such as allantoin, calcium salts, and mucopolysaccharides.

The alkaloids in any plant are referred to as "active ingredients" whose potency is stabilized by the presence of other buffers. As in human chemistry, the biochemical makeup of plants is delicate, miraculous, and complex. Chemicals which might be damaging on their own exist within both our bodies and the bodies of plants without harming us because they are offset by other chemicals. Western medicine-making focuses on isolating these alkaloids, defining as active those plant chemicals whose effects are capable of being measured by the instrumentation of western scientific methods. The drug made from the chemical formula of an isolated alkaloid often brings with it side effects that endanger the organism ingesting the substance. The less dramatic but equally important chemicals which balance the alkaloid's action and prevent side effects are often dismissively removed from synthetic formulation, perhaps because they are too subtle or volatile to be measured through western techniques.

It is interesting to note that the pyrrolizidine in comfrey exists in an organic state; the pyrrolizidine used in the laboratory studies was not organic. In general, inorganic compounds are much less easily absorbed and degraded when digested by the human body. It is both critical and ethically questioning to point out that the amount of comfrey given to the unfortunate animals tested was 50 percent of their total diet. This amount is outrageously greater than what would be ingested for medicinal or nourishing purposes. According to herbalist Adele Dawson, one would have to drink the equivalent of four cups of comfrey leaf tea each day for 140 years to be affected as the rats were affected. It is simple common sense to conclude that excessive consumption of any substance renders it poisonous.

Other tests have found only traces of pyrrolizidine in comfrey, the amount varying from plant to plant. The *American Journal of Medicine,* which reported a case of veno-occlusive liver disease from comfrey consumption, reported that the woman drank as much as ten cups of comfrey a day and a handful of tablets. As Rosemary Gladstar wisely notes, without the complete case history of these patients, it is difficult to ascertain whether comfrey was the only possible cause of liver pathology. James Duke, former U.S. Department of Agriculture botanist, calculated that wine is 144 times more cancer causing than an equal amount of comfrey tea. He used the HERP index, a scale which measures and classifies the cancer-causing potential of various substances. According to the index, comfrey has about the same cancer-causing potential as a peanut butter sandwich. I would add that nutritionally, comfrey offers quite a bit more than peanut butter, being rich in protein, calcium, iron, B vitamins, and vitamin A.

What I find significant about the comfrey controversy is that it illustrates our current reliance on external authority, here in the form of laboratory testing, for "data" which inform our health-care choices. The conflicting information disclosed through laboratory tests, as well as the questionable methods these tests employ which cause suffering to animals and do not often stage a scenario similar to what a human would engage in while working with the tested substance, awakens us to a simple fact. It is our responsibility to deeply and thoroughly investigate claims made for or against any substance being sold to us for the sake of our health. It is our task to care for ourselves by applying a healthy skepticism, a willingness to gather information, both empirically, instinctively, and intuitively, and come to our own conclusions about our health-care choices.

I am a great believer in community feedback about plants. My own information-gathering process, while it includes researching herbals, focuses on active discussion with folks I know who have had direct experience with the plant. When people tell me a plant "worked" or "didn't work," I always ask how much of the plant they used, in what form, for how long, and were they experimenting with other techniques simultaneously. I gather information by seeking out the plant; if I do not know it, I find a place it is growing, perhaps a local botanic garden, and see what the plant looks like and smells like, and how I feel around the plant or tree. If I am purchasing the herb, I buy from companies I know and trust, whose ethics I have investigated; if I am buying from the local herb store, I ask them where they have gotten the herb, and I use my nose, and my olfactory reaction to the plant, to help me decide if it is useful for my body.

I am aware that all of these methods may seem time consuming and require a sensitivity one may feel one does not possess. However, sensitivity is bequeathed to us at birth through our instincts, which respond to employment of our senses and memory. Instinct assists us in self-protection and decision-making, and can be accessed and restored with practice. My style of gathering information in relation to my health is an ongoing journey. Each organism's way of feeling out situations is unique. What is important is that one's method of assessment leads to self-trust mixed with common sense in choice-making.

The tradition of herbalism in which I trained discouraged the use of concentrated and heavily processed substances on the grounds that the further away a plant from its organic form, the more stress it incurs upon the body's digestive and absorptive channels. This idea made sense to me, for it confirmed my body's emphatic refusal to accept both food and medication offered in "extra-strength" and "convenient" form.

When one is taking an herb which has somehow been made into a pill, or powdered and stored in capsule form, one is dealing with the equivalent of a processed food. As with most mass-produced food substances, the consumer does not know who gathered the plant, from where, the conditions the plant was growing in, if it came into contact with any other substances, and how long the powder or pill was sitting around. These less-obvious criteria contribute to presence or lack of safety and potency in a preparation.

I do not mean to utterly dismiss the usefulness of these products; they have their place. Vitamin supplements have offered great relief to those undergoing chemotherapy. I myself deeply enjoy powdering herbs; grinding seeds and leaves in the mortar with my own hands invokes and links me to my ancestors, the common medicine women who tenderly prepared herbal tonics for the village folk. As all cooks know, grinding and powdering dramatically release oils and energies from deep inside the plant. However, synthesized vitamin substances are not received by the human body with the same enthusiasm and ease as vitamins from a whole food source. As an herbalist interested in medicine with vitality, I prefer to powder my herbs right before I am going to apply a powder to my gums, or to an external wound. I am suspicious of powders which have sat in gelatin capsules for an undetermined period of time; I cannot be sure of what is in them unless I have pounded the dried herb myself.

In old herbals, comfrey is lauded as a medicine chest unto itself. It has been used for centuries in England in particular, and is often called a "wonder herb." I give you the lore and wisdom of comfrey, inviting you to decide for yourself as to the safety of this herb. Every bit of information I am including here comes from my personal experience with the plant as well as the experience of persons in my community in the East Village and my relatives in Brooklyn who have benefited from the use of comfrey. The comfrey I have used for my own health and the health of those close to me has been gathered whole, wildcrafted by my own two hands, respectfully harvested from my own garden and from community gardens in upstate New York at various times of the year. It is difficult to distrust a plant you have felt warm you and strengthen you down to the bones, feeding you internal power and easing the ills of your family. If you are not prepared to look into the origins and sources of your medicine, you may want to avoid comfrey.

When comfrey leaves first peep up out of the ground, the edges of their leaves are rolled up, revealing the downy, green-gray, and veiny underside of the leaf. Each spring, small clusters of these fine young leaves often unfold near the site of the original mother plant and can be safely replanted. By midsummer, these once small offshoots thrust up into hairy, thick-stalked, six-foot-tall plants whose pearl-pink and magenta flowerbells are suckled by the bees. The regenerative nature of this plant is a prime example of the delightful hardiness of the life force.

A member of the forget-me-not tribe and the borage family, comfrey is under the dominion of the planet Saturn. Saturnian plants are considered cooling; their nature is to restrict, contract, and set limits. Astrologically, Saturn allows discipline and governs time-bound processes. As a Saturnian plant, comfrey affects the slow-growing body parts such as bones, and accomplishes a great deal of healing over time. Though seventeenth-century herbalist/astrologer Culpeper describes comfrey as cooling, and it certainly is gently contractive, I experience a deep, pervasive warmth that comforts all the mucus membranes in my gastrointestinal tract when I drink heated comfrey infusion. In the summer, I add a sprig of mint to my comfrey brew and drink it cold, its amber-colored richness feeding me green glowing strength in the form of vitamins and minerals.

Comfrey is astringent, demulcent, highly mucilaginous, and expectorant, making it a wonderful herb for soothing the lungs. Both the leaf and fall dug root of comfrey make a tasty syrup which loosens and expels phlegm from the walls of the lungs. Maud Grieves reports using comfrey for internal hemorrhage in the lungs, stomach, and bowels. The expectorant quality of comfrey is assisted by the plant's mucilage, which softens and soothes inflammation in the throat and relaxes the stomach.

Comfrey has long been considered a choice herb for working with ulcers. The demulcent leaves and roots neutralize stomach acids, coating the walls of the stomach and repairing the stomach wall with allantoin, comfrey's cell-regenerating substance. For bleeding ulcers, combine comfrey with plantain leaves *(Plantago major)* to stanch blood flow while healing the inward wound. A simple cup of comfrey tea comforts an aching stomach and wards off stomach viruses.

Comfrey, commonly called knitbone, works miraculously to speed the healing of broken bones. Several years ago my grandmother Leah, in her late eighties, fell and broke her hip. Each day my mother visited her in the hospital, she brought a quart of comfrey leaf infusion. Mom added a dropperful of comfrey root tincture to each cup my grandmother sipped. Leah's bones healed so quickly that the doctors had to reschedule her physical therapy rehabilitation to three weeks earlier than they had forecast. Culpeper remarked "and [comfrey] is special good for ruptures and broken bones; so powerful to consolidate and knit together, that if they be boiled with dissevered pieces of flesh in a pot, it will join them together again." The cell-reparative allantoin in comfrey acts almost as glue to bind that which has been broken, be it bones or epithelial tissue.

Comfrey repairs torn ligaments, cartilage, and hastens the growth of connective tissue. Sipped daily as an infusion for up to a period of several years (one or two cups a day), comfrey slowly heals old injuries which have affected joints, ligaments, cartilage, and bones and gradually strengthens weak ligaments and muscles, particularly in the knee area. A poultice of dried comfrey root powder mixed with hot water and a bit of olive oil, applied to the affected area and covered by a heating pad, penetrates into areas of tendinitis to relieve swelling and restore suppleness.

An old, single-toothed, deaf man in my community garden told me he'd had trouble with his knee for years. After accompanying me on a weed walk where I discussed comfrey, he tried it, applying a poultice to his knee for several days and eating the leaves, which he lightly steamed. His knee pain disappeared, never to return. The astringent tannins in comfrey relieve inflammation deep in the knee joint as the allantoin slowly regenerates torn cartilage. The plant's astringency reduces tissue swelling while its mucilage eases bruises. Comfrey and yarrow work well as a poultice to soothe and relieve hemorrhoids and tighten varicosities.

If the nerves have become involved due to chronic muscular spasm, I combine comfrey with flowering Saint-John's-wort for gradual deep relief. In general, I gather comfrey in late spring, when its stalks are tall and before the flowers have emerged, the plant possessing the highest concentration of allantoin at this time.

Comfrey leaves are emollient, and I often include them in facial steams mixed with lavender and rose petals. The steam opens up the lungs and brings up stuck phlegm while its green moisture penetrates into one's open pores. Hot compresses of comfrey gently encourage pliancy of the perineum during labor, ease sore nipples, and soothe the infant's umbilicus as infusion of the leaves enriches breast milk and quickens its flow. Comfrey root sitz baths keep vaginal tissues strong and supple during the menopausal years; the infusion relieves dry mouth. Rich in steroidal saponins, comfrey balances hormonal fluctuations and regulates the menstrual cycle.

Comfrey leaves and roots contain potassium, calcium, phosphorus, iron, magnesium, and cobalt. The plant is high in thiamine and riboflavin and contains vitamins C and E. Vitamin and mineral richness combined with the growth-encouraging allantoin make comfrey almost unsurpassable as a wound-healing herb. Rich in amino acids, the building blocks of protein, comfrey builds healthy bones in babies; its calcium-laden leaves keep the bones of adults, especially menopausal women, dense. Comfrey supports the bones of elders in strength and pliancy, its minerals preventing the skeletal brittleness which causes older people to slip and break their bones. Comfrey contains all the vitamins and minerals necessary for preventing backache. The leaves may be eaten raw, as a tonic in the springtime, before their surface hairs become sharp. I dip the large leaves in batter and fry them as an all-purpose nutritive meal. In parts of Ireland, comfrey was eaten as a cure for limp circulation and bloodlessness.

When treating open wounds, I do *not* use comfrey because the high protein content of the plant is a ripe breeding ground for bacteria. This same protein richness, however, is helpful for restoring healthy bacterial flora in the intestines, aiding digestion and harmonizing the internal intestinal environment which has been thrown off by the use of antibiotics or the unbalanced presence of candida albicans. Comfrey poultices are soothing to unbroken skin wounds and swellings; its moist mucilage softens boils and abseses and quickly dissolves them. When I have an open cut, I do apply comfrey root ointment to the swollen, red tissue around the mouth of the wound to soothe the hurt and encourage new cell growth.

Comfrey's clusters of drooping cuplike flowers open in late May, gracing us with pink, magenta, and blue petals which taste both sweet and gummy. The leaves, rich in potash, act as a potent soil fertilizer around the base of tomato plants. Cutting back the plants before they flower will yield several rounds of large leaves for harvesting throughout the summer. This year, I gathered armloads of flowering comfrey from a field filled with thousands of comfrey and nettle plants, all my height. At the time, I wondered if I was taking more than I needed, but my intuition guided me to persist. Later in the fall, a dancer student of mine was dropped by a fellow dancer during rehearsal; using her arm to break her fall, she tore the ligaments in her forearm. I was able to give her a shopping bag full of comfrey, as well as some root ointment, which speeded her recovery.

As an herbalist, the controversy around comfrey cautions me to refrain from using the plant with people who have damaged or sluggish livers, or women who are pregnant, though I have never had any dangerous experiences with this proud, regal herb. A gift to any garden, comfrey's deeply veined, dark-green, large leaves and cascading flowers bring joy to all eyes that rest upon them.

❧ COMFREY SALAD DRESSING

6 or 7 medium size comfrey leaves
yogurt
lemon
garlic

Chop the comfrey leaves. Place in a blender. Add two to three parts yogurt to each part comfrey leaves. Add one-half a garlic clove. Puree in the blender. Add lemon to taste.

❧ COMFREY TEMPURA

1 cup whole wheat flour
1 organic egg
pinch of sea salt
a stack full of fresh, springtime comfrey leaves
olive oil
pan
paper towels (recycled, no fragrance) and a plate

dipping sauce:
2 ounces tamari
a bit of fresh ginger root, minced
finely chopped garlic

thinly sliced scallions

½ teaspoon of organic apricot preserves

Heat the oil. Beat the egg. Dip the leaves in the egg, roll in the flour/salt mixture, and fry, turning when golden brown. Place done pieces on a plate lined with a paper towel. Cover with a paper towel and stack the fried leaves. You can use large leaves, but cook these a bit longer, so the fiberglasslike hairs on the leaves melt.

In the blender, mix the tamari and preserves. Add the chopped ginger and garlic. Before serving, lightly sprinkle scallion rings into the sauce. Dip in the cooked comfrey and enjoy.

ℰ STOMACH SOOTHING TEA

2 parts comfrey leaf

1 tsp fennel seeds

½ part comfrey root

½ part slippery elm bark

Bruise the fennel seeds with a stone. Place the herbs in a half-gallon jar. Infuse them in boiled water for four to eight hours. Reheat the infusion, and add honey to taste. The herbs all strengthen the walls of the stomach as they soothe; this concoction is wonderful for those with ulcers and is nourishing and gentle enough to be taken by nursing mothers to enrich their breast milk. If you are concerned about comfrey's effect on an infant, omit the root. If you are fearful, leave out the comfrey altogether.

RETURNING

On my September walks my eyes sweep over the ground in search of the first brightly colored fallen leaf. I always bend down and pick up this leaf, gazing deeply at its pattern, often drawing or painting its hues and pressing the leaf between the pages of a book I am reading. This lone leaf pulls me into autumn, sparking memories and expectations of cool air, brilliant color, and hot cider. That we can count on the natural world to offer us these familiar emblems of seasonal change, that they return year after year as if out of loyalty to us, gives us a precious sense of comfort and security in a world where so much is uncertain. Something in me settles down as I spy that first leaf, and I find myself gathering the light green acorns that fall to the ground, often still joined to the stem of a branch of oak leaves that have been dropped by an animal building its autumn nest.

As I walk under oak trees ringed by mounds of groundnuts that crunch beneath my shoes, I muse upon these acorns, for I know them to be a symbol of male fertility: they are often used to tip the wands of male witches. From there my thoughts wander to the god of the land, believed by the Druids to inhabit the oak. Known throughout the dark season as the lord of the shadows, this god accompanies the crone goddess as they touch all with withering, death and sleep. With pipe and flute the lord lulls all creatures to winterlong slumber; in the months of extreme cold he becomes a strong, old spirit who lives deep in the wood. Throughout the still season he guards the scattered seeds that will become the new year's field and forest.

Come spring, the lord of the wood, energized by the returning light, stirs the seed to awaken from under the ground. He transforms into the horned god, whose staglike antlers symbolize the streaming life force of the earth which courses up the forms of all creatures and bursts out the crown of the head. This vital springtime lord dances hard, leaping and landing on hoofed feet that swirl the dust up off the earth and summon all life to rise. He bends and cups a hand around each plant, whispering melodies to the reeds and grasses, breathing song into the river.

But in autumn it is an elder figure who joins the crone, who brings the shadowy long nights in which the seed lies dormant and we are coaxed into the comfort of home. In September, as the dark stretches its wings and invites us into her embrace, I find myself drawn to the what lies beneath the skins of all things. As I observe the natural world preparing for death and sleep in this month, I cannot help but notice the seeds which mature around me. Driven by curiosity, I wander around my garden, following the path of tweeting sparrows and hustling squirrels in search of seeds, ever awed by the hulls, husks, pods, and purses designed by nature to encapsulate the often tiny blueprint of each green species.

Staining the knees of my jeans as I kneel, I peer under the brim of violet's heart-shaped, now fading leaves, uncovering the star-shaped capsule at the base of its stem, each slit point bearing rows of black, round balls. Craning my neck up to the empress tree, I memorize the oval hull which encloses the seeds. Come February, each husk will split and release a brown, notched elliptical disc, cleft as a vulva; the burst seed capsules will lie like castanets along the ground. Thrusting my hand into the shadowy green forest of the yew bush, I pull a berry, its red, jellied flesh protecting the seed, poison to humans, at its core.

Within each form of life on earth is a vessel, seen or unseen, that carries the regenerative potential of the species. Indeed, the number of seeds and the unique shapes that nature provides to each life form for its continuance is staggering. Seeds are the promise of return gifted to us as death and hibernation settle over the land. Gathering, separating, and drying the seeds of plants ingrains in us the deep certainty of rebirth. The firm, internal knowing this act brings sustains us as we approach and enter the time of the dark, freeing us to embrace this contemplative time and to be cradled in its fertile blackness.

During September, on the equinox or when the moon is waning, buy an organic fall squash. With a sharp knife, cut it lengthwise, exposing its seed bearing center. With a spoon or by hand, scoop out the seeds and place them in a colander. Place the halves of squash face down in a shallow pan, pour in about a one-quarter inch of water and bake them in a 350° oven for about an hour. After awhile, the house will be filled with a rich, sweet aroma.

As the squash cooks, pour cool water over the seeds, stirring them around and around with your fingers. The seeds possess a slippery coating and are connected to the central cavity of the squash by thin strands of flesh. Continue to rinse and stir the seeds with the water, absorbing yourself in the task, in your own way becoming present to the miracle of the seed. As you stir, sense within you the place where seeds of new life live. Gently pour and stir until all the pulp and viscous coating is gone from the seeds. When you are done, lay the seeds on a paper towel, place them in a spot where they will be undisturbed. Let them dry.

When the squash is done, drizzle butter and cinammon over it and eat its plump innards. Though its flesh has now become yours, its sweet potential lives in the seeds you have carefully preserved. Days later, when the seeds have dried, peel them off the towel, place them in a pouch or envelope and tuck them into a dark, warm place, keeping them hidden until spring. As the inward season progresses, return in your mind to the seeds, and where you have hidden them. You may want to periodically take out and hold the pouch in which you have laid the seeds, but do not remove them from their dark home. Rest in the confident truth that multitudinous seeds of creativity and life live unborn within you, and in their time, and from the same mysterious birthplace as the returning spring, they will enter this world.

OCTOBER

Slowing, Rooting, Releasing

OCTOBER ARRIVES, BEARING a secret. Children already know this secret, for in keeping with their elfin bodies, they live and move close to the ground, where they inhale the sweet rot of fallen leaves and warm steam rises out of the decay to chase the chill from their cheeks. I learned the secret from a maple tree with sixty hoops in its black, rain-glistened trunk and a huge knob scarred with grooves bulging from its middle. As a child with eyes that scoured the ground in search of wonder, my small hands caressed the rough gall which swelled from the waistline of this tree, certain it was a doorknocker hiding a portal to the world inside the maple. The trails of thick, twisted roots that stretched from the base of the tree formed a stepstool upon which I could stand and touch the burl in the hopes of gaining entrance into the maple. The small arroyos between the roots were inhabited by brown-bodied ants and several families of beige-capped mushrooms arranged in rings.

In spring, bouquets of lime green buds dropped from the maple's branches, which began their arch from the trunk some fifty feet above my head. In fall, these leaves flamed pomegranate-red, lemon and rust as they dropped at times swiftly, more often slowly to the sidewalk. I squinted into the distance: the ground seemed strewn with small, motionless animal bodies. Why, I wondered, did the maples and oaks shake their leaves to the ground in the first place? I dropped my head back, my eyes climbing the maple's trunk to its highest branch in search of an answer. The maple, however, remained silent.

One late October afternoon, my senses hungry for the fresh scent that follows an October downpour, I leashed up my dog and went out for a stroll. As he sniffed and stiffened his tail at the bark of one thin sapling, I inhaled deep draughts of rain-sweetened, cool air and peered absently into the distance. In the night, the pelting rain had flattened the bright leaves to the ground. As the small pools in their centers evaporated, the leaf-edges began to curl and peel off the cement. From where I stood, each leaf looked like an ear pressed to the earth. As I stared at these scattered ears, I heard a voice ricochet off the walls of my skull, asking: "why do the trees shake their leaves to the ground in the first place?" A deep rumbling laugh rose up behind me. I whirled around, inadvertently wrapping my ankles with the dog's leash. I cocked my head, puzzled. Only the maple was at my back. I shrugged, turned to continue, and—again, the vibrating laugh. A shiver rose up my back. This time, I did not turn around.

The laughter was followed by a voice that scratched like wind through dead, dull-brown leaves barely hanging from the mother branch. "The answer," the voice hissed and creaked. "is in these leaf-ears that now cleave to the ground. They remind us . . ." the voice paused, and exhaled heavily, whistling as it inhaled another breath. "They remind us that the time of silence now rises from below, elongating itself like a shadow over the ground. The season where quiet blooms and we tilt our ears like leaves toward the hushed air and earth draws near. If we do this, the north winter wind and the cold which rides the back of the silence will bring voices. The voices of those we wish to remember and the voices of all not yet born. But first," the speaker whispered, its speech slipping back to its silent source, "first you must be as these leaves. You must do what the leaves now do." The voice was gone.

A gust of wind tossed the leaves upward and sent them skipping along the sidewalk. My dog's pink tongue licked the young tree's bark. Somewhat stunned and pensive, I pulled on his leash and turned homeward. So this was the secret, I thought as I hurried home, the rising quarter moon glowing and slashed by charcoal branches forking across the delphinium sky. *You must do as the leaves now do.*

All that night the question thrust itself at me like an excited child bursting into the room: what do the leaves do? Finally, I put my work aside; pouring myself a cup of sassafras-leaf tea, I sat by the window, in view of the copper bark of our backyard cherry and gave my attention to answering.

The subtle spice of sassafras steam stroked my sinuses as I sipped and mused. What do I know of the habits of leaves? What does it mean, as the maple pronounced, to be as the leaves? I rocked in my chair and thought hard. I know that they choose as they age to exchange the green cloak of youth for the vermillion, salmon, and mauve of the sky at sunset. I see that in their time, leaves release their hold on the tree, swinging like a pendulum back and forth on currents of air, then caught and suspended by the zigzag of branches or settling mutely on the ground. Leaves of oak, maple, sassafras, barberry, gingko, and sycamore drape over the earth like a hide, warming and nourishing the ground even in death. As their numbers mount, the leaf-pelt thickens, becoming prize matter for creatures that roam thicket, field, and air in search of winter shelter. The pungent beauty of leaves intensifies as they age; at each ledge of decay they gracefully serve the circle of beings and environ they inhabit. Yes, I concluded, there are many habits the green nations invite us to follow as they shed their summer garb and prepare for the season of bitter winds, ice, and snow.

SLOWING

In October the crone's skin turns translucent, the slowing pulse of life revealed in the rivulets of arteries and veins beneath her fist that grasps the branch and shakes the leaves loose. Trailing her cloak across the landscape, she unravels the hem of natural laws which influence bounty, checking summer's rampant flow of growth. In fairy tales the crone is a shapeshifter, assuming the form of owls, blackbirds, children, young men, and rosebushes, through her guises gaining entrance into all realms. Her task is to restore balance, be that by bringing death, justice, birth, or blessing into the domains she visits. The crone's skill of moving deftly between the province made solely of spirit and the world of matter is made available to humans at this turn of the year, when the membrane between these two worlds grows as thin as the dying leaf and the language of the over- and underworlds become intelligible to the human ear.

Weaver of change, and bringer of death, the crone sleeps in the wrinkled red berry, the bare branch that flashes across our vision as we stare into May's flowering hawthorn. Though her death touch may be swift or slow, compassion rather than cruelty is her companion. The crone's fingertips close the lids of the mortally wounded deer; plant by plant she cups her palms around the seed-heavy crowns of the grasses, her warm breath propelling the moist life of the plant into the root, leaving its aerial parts hollow and wizened. The life force nestles and dips into a hidden place, a world of mystery from which it grows young and rises renewed come spring.

Before each act which ends life, the crone carefully considers how a particular death will affect the pattern of the natural world. She encircles each creature, uttering the sound which halts the growth cycle and calls bareness, deep sleep, dormancy, and change. The leaves she has touched remind us that death can be breathtaking and inspiring when the moment of letting go comes in its proper course. As fallen leaves grow quiet, we too can slow and settle ourselves down, creating or finding an inner ground; in this soil, we can prepare for ourselves a bed we can dream in, tuning our rhythm to that of the October earth which begins to harden and draw its heat and substance inward and downward. Following the pattern of the trees, we slowly and steadily shed our outer ornaments, thickening our skins like tree bark and pulling our energies within.

ROOTING

The icy exhalation of the crone rings the moon in an iridescent glimmer and brings a sudden first frost which alerts the green nations to the hovering winter. Overnight, the life force of the plants plummets below ground, deserting the topside world and traveling the labyrinthian pathways of roots and rhizomes which form the map of the underground. As

October unfolds, our green allies focus the source of their nourishment away from the sun, rain, and air toward the earth, fattening their roots with minerals and starches pulled from the plant's uppermost parts, the earth and the water in the soil.

Unlike the mobile, wind-borne nutrients of carbon dioxide and sun radiance which the plant catches by offering a large, above-ground surface area of stem, leaf, and flower, the nutritive mineral salts below ground are still. In order to suckle this underground food, plants develop elaborate mazes of roots, their generous girth offering more body surface to the touch of the soil. In this manner, the roots directly absorb nutrients from the earth through the contact of their root skin and root hairs with the ground.

In addition to its absorptive capacity, the root anchors the plant to the ground, holding it firm in the face of storms and protecting its life in situations where the exposed plant body is torn and destroyed. In the warmer months, the root of the plant also acts as a bridge, conducting nutrients to the stem of the plant and the inner bark of trees. In October, as winter looms, roots also serve as a storage chamber, preserving food for the plant's dormant period in the form of starch. For the herbalist, October and November are optimal months for garnering potent physical and magical root medicine from the plants as well as harnessing starches and sugars which keep us nourished through green-slim winter months.

When one gathers roots one is giving death. And so one must become the crone, carefully considering the effect of the act upon the environment. One must uproot flippancy, hurry, or casualness from the ground of one's own mind before taking trowel or spade in hand. Then one must, with certainty and clarity, be able to see as the crone sees, how this death will create the space for new life. One must press one's ears to the ground of mystery, listening for the voice of the plant which calls the root digger toward it to gather its flesh. Medicines made with such attentiveness often initiate healing in both the body and spirit.

The act of mindful root digging builds concentration and nurtures a deep respect for the plants who give their power for the sake of human healing. Using small hand tools and attempting to pull the root out whole, though it increases the time spent gathering a single root, develops a patience and persistence which alters the rhythm out of which we dance our life. An attitude of partnership with the plant and with unseen forces is required to separate an anchored root from its mother soil without violence. As our hands and trowel circle round and round to reveal and loosen the root, our eyes roam this hidden plant body as one would the shape and skin of a lover, to learn its ways and needs, the story of strength and vulnerability detailed in its scars.

Much like Persephone and her six pomegranate seeds, because roots have eaten the riveted underground nutrients, they become forever kin to this dark, other world. And as we eat of these roots, during the dark months of the year we grow a skin that allows us to traverse this expansive, hidden terrain, becoming privy to the messages of all that one discovers in the underworld realm. The autumn and winter heart of this cavernous place beats slow and deep, and all who become attuned to the rhythm found in the still time learn to savor the snap of twigs and the scent of birch smoke, to penetrate the meaning-filled essence of the sights and sounds that compose the numerous, precise activities of late fall.

While today we use spades and forks to unearth roots, at other times there have been bones and bird claws, talons, beaks, and incantations used by humans to separate root from soil. If they have learned their craft soulfully, today's wildcrafters and herbalists will know that each plant has a way it likes to be taken and may, if asked, guide the digger to carry out its specific instructions. As we quiet our thinking, the murmuring of the plants becomes audible, and the wish of the plant regarding its harvesting may be apprehended.

Several years ago, I drove out to Connecticut for a summer wedding. The eve of the wedding, the groom's half-brother and I stayed up into the night, our conversation interrupted only occasionally by the hoot of barred owls. As we crossed the threshold from the kitchen to the living room with our mugs of tea, I commented on the invisible curtain which seemed to brush my face as we passed from room to room. He began to whisper stories of the house's origins, offering the advanced age and history of the town nearby, of the witches hunted there, and how this house which he had grown up in still seemed to be peopled with spirits.

As he spilled his tales, the hair on my body became electric, poised excitedly and fearfully for contact with unseen forces. Rain beat the screens of the porch I was to sleep in. A thick green sweetness curled into the room through its fine grids. Placing a candle he had made himself by my bedside table, the brother bid me good night and retreated to his attic loft, where he sealed himself in to carve a wedding candle for the bride and groom.

I awoke only briefly in the night, to the sound of a racoon rubbing its muzzle against the door. By morning the rain had emptied itself, but the sky was white with clouds. We had hoped for a beautiful day, and I circled the thirteen apple trees in the grove where the wedding was to be held, chanting a homemade rhyme calling to the sun. The small orchard was surrounded by a hedgerow of rhododendrons and blossoming elder trees which I skirted, collecting flowers for the wreaths of the betrothed couple. My hands full of elder, rosemary, and lavender, I entered the stand of pine trees, my eyes combing the ground for fallen evergreen branches to bend into fragrant circlets.

The tall pines formed a cathedral under which my body relaxed and released its city tension. I sank down on a tree root, my skirt filled with flowers. Leaning my head against the tree trunk, I narrowed my eyes to slits and wished myself invisible to the other guests. As I rested, I noticed dozens of young poke plants around each tree. Extremely stimulating to the immune system and used with discretion by seasoned herbalists, I often saw *Phytolacca americana* in New York City, its thick, magenta stems and striated roots too entrenched in the earth to dig out with a spade. But these young plants! Perhaps they would come more easily, though they would be less potent in the July heat than after the first frost. I decided to make a bit of oil which would work more gently than a mature, fall dug root.

I asked the plants. They invited me to return after the ceremony. Hours later, I borrowed a spade from the garage and disappeared again into the canopy of pine. Leaning my shovel against a tree trunk, I walked from poke to poke, bending down and praying for a plant to give me a signal that it was willing to become medicine. I passed by a second, third, and fourth poke root. Then I turned in another direction, toward a plant which seemed to draw my head around. As I approached it I felt something in the poke leap in my direction. My bones told me that this plant had offered itself. Barehanded, I drew its stem and leaves to one side, parting it carefully as one would a child's hair, in order to examine the crown where stem and root became the other. I knew the crowns of *Phytolacca americana* could be replanted and the poke would continue to grow. I grasped my hand around the crown of the root to sense the size and depth of it. As I held the poke, its foot long root slid out of the earth, whole, into my hand.

I stood dumbfounded, the root in my palm. I had not even pulled. The plant had given itself to me in a manner I had only read about, in a moment when I had forsaken expectation, when I happened to be practicing respect in my medicine making. I held the root up to the sunlight, which by noon had begun to to burn through the chalky sky. The base itself began as a broad crown which forked into a pair of taproots that plaited around one another at their thickest points and remained singular at their slender tips. Held away from me, the ivory root resembled thighs entwined in a lovers' embrace. The entire root matched the length of my elbow to middle finger.

I recalled the root doctors of the south, who sewed pouches to carry specific roots they gathered and charmed, selling the individually prepared packets as powerful medicine to be tucked into the pocket and worn by a client to ward off evil, prevent disloyalty, increase fertility, or banish another black magician's work. I decided to prepare the poke root as a gift to the wedding couple. Disappearing into the house, I found the empty box of another present which had been unwrapped and returned outside, layering it with the earth that had surrounded the root. Carefully laying the root upon its bed, I asked poke to strengthen the immunity of the couple to divisive influences. I jotted a little note explaining my gift, and placed the box on the table amidst the growing pile of giftwrapped boxes. Satisfied, I returned to the pines, filled the gap of earth with soil and covered it with pine needles, thanking poke for this experience.

The teachings and medicine of the green nations is infinite, spontaneous, and unusual, often uniquely suited to the person engaging with the plant. Working with roots is effortful, but I cherish the subtle and profound nourishment, sensual delight, and wisdom this work brings. And as our labor to unearth roots is slow and rich, so is the pace of root medicine as it grasps hold of and lodges within our bodies.

Traditional Chinese medicine, which for thousands of years has explored and sought to understand the physical and energetic medicine healing power brought to us in the form of food, considers root vegetables robust forces of chi (life force) for the human body. Roots expand our reservoir of vivacity, widening our foundational energy and instilling us with solidity, increasing our connection with the earth.

I believe roots are best used in herbal medicine to reach the root causes of syndromes, chronic problems, and dis-eases, to locate, transform, or uproot the source of the disturbance and to bring minerals and vitamins into the bloodstream that restore tired organs and overworked systems. The easily assimilable organic composition of vitamins and minerals housed in the plant's late fall and early spring roots allow our cells to receive powerful nutrition, much in the way rootlets and root hairs draw out the minerals, salts and waters from the medicine we have imbibed. Certain plants contain specific alkaloids which, over time, challenge deeply entrenched organ and system patterns and replace them with the ancient imprint of natural strength with which these organs were originally imbued.

The actions of absorption, anchoring, conduction, and storage which are the skill of the roots are a signature of their pull toward strengthening the human organs and body systems which function in a similar way. Without even knowing about particular roots one could intuit, for example, that the gall bladder, which stores bile, the lymphatic system, which conducts wastes, the bloodstream, which conducts nutrients, waste, hormones, and other chemicals, and the small intestine, which absorbs nutrients, would be some of the organs and systems enhanced and rejuvenated by the use of root medicine. Roots which grow near streams might indicate their power on both the liquids and conduits of the body, and their ability to increase flow where stagnation and blockage has occurred. Herbs that thrust their taproots deep into the soil can find their way into deeply clutching dis-ease, search out, and nurture the hidden ground of health within the body that has been eclipsed by illness.

The plant I have chosen for October has been greatly revered around the world for many centuries. Its root is used extensively by the Chinese in food, where it is called *gobo,* and grows as a tenacious weed near streams, construction sites, forest, and open field. The root of this plant will circumnavigate stones in the earth and continue to plunge downward in search of nourishment, reaching depths of four feet. A plant that nurtures persistence, indeed! This plant dives into the foundation of one's being, pulling out what has been gasping for breath and stifling within, searching for, feeding, and bringing to light reservoirs of inner strength that lay curled and sleeping within the shadowy corners of the psychic and physical body. This plant is the sweet, succulent, mighty burdock.

BURDOCK *(Arctium lappa)*

Burdock's botanical name, *Arctium lappa,* is derived from the greek *arctos,* meaning bear, and the Celtic *llap,* meaning hand, or to seize. These words refer to the infamous round seed pouches of burdock, covered in prickly hooks which seize the clothing, fur, and hair of all bodies grazing past burdock's mature, brown burrs. The plant propagates far and wide by hitching a ride on sheep, dogs, humans, and cows, spreading its medicine through countryside and city lot. Velcro fasteners were originally patterned upon the burrs of *Arctium,* and the seeds inside are potent medicine. Some of burdock's amusing folk names are beggar's buttons, stick tight, cockle burr, clotbur, and batweed. As those who have wandered through patches of burdock in autumn know, to bend over a burr as one gathers is to quite likely be caught in the buttocks by the burrs of another burdock plant. I make sure to leave my favorite sweater at home when on a burdock field trip, as plucking the fiberglass-like hairs out of the wool is best left to fairies and dwarves specializing in accomplishing impossible tasks during the wee hours of morning.

Fresh burdock root is nutritive; the fall-dug root of first-year plants and spring-dug roots of second-year plants are rich in vitamins and minerals. A biennial plant with a two-year life cycle, burdock sends its starches and sugars down to the root to be preserved as winter passes overground. During its second year, burdock grows a stalk through which it thrusts energy, nutrition, and medicine into the flowers and fruits in order to propagate itself. Dig up the root of a second year plant after its flowers have opened and you will find a dead, woody stalk, too fibrous for eating. The root of the first-year plant is a succulent, earthy delicacy that conjures up the flavor of Jerusalem artichokes.

Burdock root is high in iron, magnesium, calcium, thiamine, potassium, and carotenes expressed as vitamin A. The fresh root contains enough vitamin C to be included in older herbals as a preventative and curative for the deficiency. Burdock root is also rich in trace minerals such as selenium, manganese, phosphorus, and chromium, and contains fiber, mucilage, and a high amount of inulin. Frequent use of burdock as a food increases one's groundedness, physical power, emotional equilibrium, and glandular and immune system health. Burdock's tonic effect on almost every system in the body contributes to effects such as sexual vitality, longevity, and freedom from cancer. Marinating burdock in vinegar and adding to the salad even once a week will increase energy and provide balance, particularly to those with sugar cravings. Burdock, used as a food, is a superb ally for those with hypoglycemia.

One fall day I was in Central Park in search of burdock with a student I loved for his ability to take sensual pleasure in the daily acts of self-care such as eating. We rolled up our shirtsleeves and dug with our small trowels (it is illegal to dig in the park). While I know internal use of burdock affects the sweat glands, digging a foot-long root with two hand tools was enough to begin that action! As we persevered through the labor of our digging, the sweet, pungent smell of burdock rose in the air between us, prompting a salivary response in both our mouths. By the time we had unearthed the root, my hypoglycemic tendency toward sudden, ravenous hunger had set in. I was starving, and we had brought water as our only food. Taking turns, we brushed most of the dirt off the young root so that our mouths would not get gritty. Inhaling its sweet, earthy scent, we bathed the root in spring water and shared bites of burdock between us.

I will never forget the immediate relief from hunger that I felt. Though we shared only a single, small root and my belly had certainly not been fed a full dinner, I felt completely satiated, strengthened, and energetically renewed. My body had received a treasure chest of vitamins and minerals which quieted and transformed not only my gnawing hunger but gave me the gift of feeling the deeply physical sensation of satisfaction brought by burdock's optimum nutrition. I felt invigorated to the point of leaping. As we pushed the soil we had unearthed back into place and patted the mound of soil in thanks, not only my stomach but my soul was satiated.

Burdock is considered to be a cooling herb, favored by herbalists for hot conditions and balancing those of stormy temperament. My personal experience, however, is that while burdock may cool the reflexes of the hot-natured, it slowly and skillfully draws to the surface hidden passion and anger for those who tend to keep the fiery side deep within. While burdock nourishes the glandular and immune system and slowly alters the strength of these systems, the tincture is also known for drawing out fluids: sweat, oil, menstrual flow, inflammation, infection, and urine. Wherever fluids are blocked or flow has dwindled to trickling proportions, burdock's hand reaches in and finds the source from which new liquids can flow, coaxing fluids to the surface of the body, bringing the moisture that renews life.

Burdock's rejuvenative skills lead me to recommend the root for those whose creative or sexual rivers seem to be running dry. The fresh root is available in most organic health food stores, and is identifiable by its earthy, sweet aroma, dull brown color, and sturdy, thick root. Burdock restores tired kidneys and liver, allowing them to better filter the blood and urine. In the liver, burdock encourages digestive and hormonal secretions which energize the intestines and wake up all the glands, moistening our sexuality and balancing sugar in the blood. The fresh root is a gentle laxative and carminative.

Burdock loves to work in partnership; combined with dandelion root, this herb rejuvenates digestion and rebuilds the liver. Alcohol extract of burdock and dandelion work beautifully as a fall tonic taken for a period of six weeks, three times a day, during which they offer their secrets of how to store energy for the winter time. Burdock and echinacea *(Echinacea angustifolia)* join hands to uproot recurrent viral and bacterial infection, such as herpes; the hot pain of genital herpes sores can be eased by poultices of freshly grated burdock root as the burdock/echinacea combination, taken internally, slowly heal the herpes. Burdock gradually alters chronic venereal infection and slow-growing viruses and cancers.

Burdock is often referred to in older herbals as an alterative, blood-purifying herb. Unlike stimulating herbs, which give quick, sometimes surface results by dramatically appearing to "cleanse" the body of impurities, burdock is an herb better understood by those accustomed to treading slow paths toward transformation. The root's style is almost tortoiselike as it patiently wades through tired organs, pulling poisons, chemical residues, and contaminants which slow down the lymphatic, digestive, and urinary organs that work with fluids. Burdock is also known for sometimes causing a "healing crisis," magnifying the symptoms of dis-ease as it dives deep to dismantle the root cause of illness.

Burdock has a particular affinity for the skin, uprooting the source of skin disturbances such as psoriasis, eczema, and acne. The seeds of burdock are used by most herbalists to affect changes in the skin, but I find the fresh root can be greatly relieving as well. A poultice of fresh, grated burdock root greatly soothes the weeping, cracked skin that accompanies raging eczema. Burdock seed oil or ointment is best used when the eczema is dry, and is effective for psoriasis in the scalp. The oil is a nourishing tonic to the hair follicles and is helpful for hair loss. A facial steam of burdock-seed infusion loosens, opens, and clears blackheads from the face. An infusion of burdock by itself or mixed with one or two other skin-healing herbs, such as nettles, red clover, or oatstraw, drunk in the same biennial cycle as the plant, will alter entrenched imbalances which express themselves through the skin. This shift may be assisted by changes in one's diet.

Burdock-seed tincture, in conjunction with poultices of the bruised leaf, help with chronic joint and skin problems. Herbalist Susun Weed notes that by increasing the output of uric acid, burdock seed prevents gout. It strongly affects the urinary tract, acting as a diuretic (the fresh root causing immediate response), easing edema, strengthening the bladder, and toning the urinary tract. The plant's demulcent abilities soothe the urinary tract and respiratory passages and moisten the intestines as well, strengthening digestion and preserving peristaltic continuity for those whose intestinal muscles have weakened from lack of food.

Burdock seed in particular eases chronic cystitis, reducing inflammation and increasing the flow of urine. Its cooling abilities are helpful when urine is burning hot and acute infection is present. Sipping cold infusion hastens the seed's cooling action. Burdock-seed tincture and infusion is helpful for women in the last months of pregnancy, when they are sometimes troubled by water retention. Native Cherokee women used burdock root to strengthen the womb before the birth and to give them stamina for labor; following birth they used the root to heal prolapse and restore vigor.

The first burdock I was introduced to had two-foot long leaves with wavy edges and a white, downy underside. A beginning herbalist, I did not know how I would ever tell the difference between a comfrey leaf and a burdock leaf. A teacher suggested I gently touch the leaf, rubbing it between my thumb and forefinger, and then taste my thumb. I was shocked by the bitterness of the leaf's oil that clung to my skin. It was that clean, bitter taste which sets the mouth's digestive juices to work and signals to us the plant's affinity for the liver and gastrointestinal tract. Bruised burdock leaves cool and ease the pain of sprains, wounds, broken bones, and many hot conditions, such as boils, skin ulcers, burns, and poison ivy. It is the bitter leaf which encourages the sweat and oil glands, promoting perspiration and menstrual flow. Burdock-leaf tea relieves the liver and headaches caused by liver torpor, quieting and cooling lingering coughs and festering anger.

Try carrying a pouch of root which you can hold in moments—often premenstrual ones—where you feel your anger may rise and either explode or implode. Send the heat of your anger through your arm into the root pouch and watch your anger drain and cool. If stronger medicine is needed, dig some roots yourself. The act of digging is superb for channeling rage into the earth, which respects, accepts, and transforms it into the fire of action and growth.

℮ AUTUMN GROUNDING ROOT TONIC TEA

2 parts burdock root and dandelion root
½ part licorice root
water
a pot

Use enough root to cover the bottom of your pot. Fill with water. The less water you use and the more you simmer the herbs, the more potent and possibly bitter the mixture will be. I use about one part herb to three parts water, letting the brew simmer for an hour. If I have leftover tea, I leave it on the stove and keep reheating the mixture, adding more water to dilute the mixture.

℮ BURDOCK ROOT EXTRACT

fresh burdock root
100 proof vodka
a jar

Chop the burdock and fill the jar completely with it, leaving as little air-space as possible. Add the vodka to the top, cap, and leave for six weeks. Over the six weeks you may have to top off the mixture. The white sediment that settles in the bottom of the jar is the precious, starchy inulin, and not mold. When you strain your extract through cheesecloth after six weeks, be sure you use the white sediment in your medicine.

℮ BURDOCK GRAVY

2 large, fresh burdock roots (at least 1 foot long each)
2 onions
whole wheat flour
olive oil

Slice the burdock into two-inch long strips. Slice the onion. Sauté both in olive oil. Add in whole wheat flour to coat the vegetables until the smell is toasty, making a roux. Add hot water until you have a thick consistency, and cook until burdock is soft. This thick gravy is wonderful with sauted mushrooms over rice.

RELEASING

During the time when all humans participated in gleaning subsistence from the earth, the last day of October marked the shift from the agriculturally fertile seasons into those months where hunting served as the people's most immediate source of food. In the Celtic lunar calendar, this month was the last of thirteen moons; the eve of the newborn year was called All-Hallow's eve, or Old-Year's night. Foods that continued to grow after Halloween were left in the fields; farmers relinquished control of the land, releasing their claim on the fruits of the autumn harvest, offering all that flourished beyond this day into the divine domain of the goddess and god as well as the ancestral dead for these forces to use in their own way.

The countryside folk held to the belief that through the whole month of October, as the lush face of the land faded into somber hues of grey and brown and much green life became skeletal, the veil which separated the spirit world from the corporeal realm became thinner and thinner. On Halloween night, this transparency peaked, allowing the spirits of the dead to slip through the boundaries that screened them from the world of matter and fly over the earth, bringing whispers of warning and hope to their living relatives. The custom of masquerading and trick or treating arose to confuse prankster spirits who might be afoot this night, bent on tricking the naive or unprotected.

If we imagine the strenuous, deeply physical work of planting and harvesting most folk engaged in from spring to late fall, it is no wonder that a mischief-making festival such as Halloween was created—it no doubt lightened the load borne by country folk during the earth's fertile months.

Halloween also marks a momentous turn on the wheel of the year. The twenty-four hours of October 31, and midnight especially, hang between the old and the new year, noosed by a slender tether to calendars calculated by those of rational mind. The day and eve of Old Year's night belong neither to the land of the living nor to the land of the dead, both to the time of endings and the time of beginnings, suspended outside of human-made concepts and laws. Intentions, declarations, wishes, and desires spoken at this time carry great power, for both the secular anchors which fix our sense of time and the elemental laws by which we are bound are relaxed. On this night, what we ask, invoke, and name reverberates throughout all time and all worlds, initiating vast changes in our lives.

Halloween's modern preoccupation with open graves out of which the dead emerge is a remnant of a ritual pilgrimage into the realm of the underworld which our cycle-sensitive ancestors knew was best undertaken on this mysterious eve. In these ancient teaching tales, one was summoned to descent by her or his own heart, stirred to compassionate action by an ability to hear the voices of lost, suffering spirits wandering about in the shadows.

As the journeyer began the quest, she or he was watched over by an elder guardian who waited at the entrance to the underworld, keeping the pilgrim linked to life through the watchkeeper's presence and prayers. At each portal of descent, the journeyer laid aside exterior ornaments of power, layer by layer revealing their true vulnerability. Though these crying spirits were fearful in their pain, by gathering the courage to embrace and soothe the ache of these souls, the pilgrim gained power and won the right of passage back into the topside world.

If we are listening, on Halloween the mournful cries of lost and wandering spirits may call us to this difficult, fruit-bearing pilgrimage into the shadows of our own psyche. As autumn deepens, the growing bareness of the trees and sparse landscape may magnify our inner barrenness, bringing up old grief that demands we dive into its waters. Thus we render death and loss sacred and honorable in an age which denies its existence.

As the old women of the villages once did, on All Hallow's eve we may wrap ourselves in the long cloak of the night, huddle around a warm fire, and keen and moan to our ancestors for all we have lost. On Halloween night, it is the crone and the lord of the shadows who act as guardians as we pass through the pain of our losses. Releasing our grief, we make room for joy to abound in the new year. And on this night, we return the land to the arms of the elder gods and goddesses, passing through the threshold from the season of activity to the season of contemplation.

As the ancient journeyer removed her or his robes to descend into the underworld, on Halloween night we relinquish to the fire all we are ready to shed, that we may come newborn and lightened to the new year. The fire burned on All Hallow's eve is no ordinary fire; it is kindled with concentration and intent, prepared with special herbs and woods believed to enhance future vision and to carry the powers of destruction and regeneration. Halloween's fire burns to recieve that which we are ready to release, in order to clear a path, to engender a ground ripe and receptive to the invisible, first cycle of seed planting: the season of preconception. The following ritual can be done in a solitary setting; however, the presence of others as we give voice to the habits and situations we intend to release forms a powerful energy of witness which encourages us to follow through on our utterances.

Sometime in October, find a park, garden, or preserve where the leaves are not raked, where you can amble through rustling piles of oak and maple leaves and muse on the year which has passed. Nature's essential calmness acts as a refuge, helping us to reinhabit ourselves fully so we can clearly discern what to offer the fire on Halloween night. Do not overburden yourself by choosing to "permanently" release a deeply entrenched habit or long-standing difficult situation. For when we call upon nature to assist us we can be sure that what we ask to shed will leave us in ever-widening spirals, for that is the underlying pattern of the natural world. Old Year's night is also a suitable time to ask the fire for a gift of fulfillment, so give some time also to asking your heart what would bring you happiness.

When you have attained clarity on these matters, search out a mature, white birch tree, one whose outer bark curls like a tongue. Birch is the tree of beginnings, and will make certain that whatever you cast into the fire will be replaced by new birth and tender growth. Asking the tree for permission first, firmly pull the curled edges of betula's outer bark, gathering enough to write your request upon. Don't forget to inhale the sweet smell of death exuded by the leaves; you may want to stuff your pockets with some dry leaves to toss into the fire. If you live in a city where the buildings have hidden the trees, you may use paper to write upon, and use a single candle as your torch rather than a flaming cauldron.

Return home for Halloween night, remembering to have some chocolate or candy on hand for the trick or treaters. You never know when a magical spirit will show up at your door in the guise of a child. After the day has turned to night, you may begin to prepare a table with a dark cloth and some candles, a fire resistant bowl, and some matches. Place mementos or photos from relatives who have passed over on the table as well as some food for the traveling spirits who wander this night. Write the words of that which you are releasing on the salmon colored side of the birch bark, or on your paper, and set the paper on the table.

Extinguishing all the lights in the room, sit in silence until you can no longer distinguish the edges of your body. Listen for the first sound of the otherworld, which is a quiet laden with the excitement of possibility. After you have honored the silence, you may call the names of your ancestors as witnesses to this rite. If you are with others, let each person present speak the name of a deceased relative whom they loved. Light the fire, tossing in dried leaves to help it ignite. If you are using a single candle, kindle it now. When the fire is blazing, stand before the flame or flames, inhaling the sharp-edged transformational essence of fire into your belly. When you begin to feel warm, ask the fire and your ancestors to assist you in your quest to release that which is ready to be shed. Then toss the written symbol into the flames. If you are holding your words to the single candle, have a small container nearby in which to place the ashes.

The fire may easily catch hold of the bark, flaming strongly for a few moments before ebbing; or it may take some time to catch the edge of the bark and will burn slowly, without much bright flame as the bark becomes cinders. When the fire is at its brightest, name aloud your heart's desire, beseeching the flames to bring you fulfillment of your dreams.

Over the years I have found that whatever I name aloud as my desire on this night will surely come to pass; perhaps because the veil between worlds is so thin that the spirits benevolent to humankind hear our need as loud as thunder.

When all have had their turn, and the fire has cooled, gather the ashes and bury them in the ground on the first of November. If you have a garden, you may save the ashes to sprinkle over the ground at spring's first planting. When the ritual is done, pass around food and wine in honor of the birth of the season of mystery. The season of the dark has just begun, with many hidden treasures to uncover, and many secrets yet to come.

THE THIRTEENTH MONTH

∾

Pausing

ONCE UPON A time, Halloween, All Soul's Day, and the Day of the Dead were considered a three-day month that stood apart from the rest of the year. Freeing the passage of three sunrises and sunsets from the written calendar added to the otherworldly feel of this triad of days. Indeed, unbound from a predictable, calendric rhythm, these three days inspired devotion to the unknowable and invisible, the chaotic and surprising.

In this time, where in many areas of dominant culture we see a scientific quest to unveil and conquer the mysteries of birth and death, where technology offers us instant access to information but has little to satisfy our hunger for true human connectedness, using these three days to pause and immerse ourselves in timelessness and not-knowing, can perhaps begin to expand our palette of responses to the unknown, replacing our fear with wonder as we bravely acquaint ourselves with the floating cycle of the void.

Pausing exists in the most basic rhythms of nature. If we lie by the ocean and listen to the sound of the waves crashing against the shore, we will hear not only the thunderous rush and retreat of the tide but also the stillness which inhabits the space between these extraordinary waxing and waning forces. Our human breath pattern, and perhaps the breathing pattern of other creatures, echoes the ocean's tidal inhalation and exhalation. If we listen to ourselves breathe, we will encounter a still space which exists between the outward and inward flow of our breath, during which our body savors the nourishment it has drawn from the air.

The natural habit of the body to take into itself nutrition during the pause of breath cycle suggest that any moment of pause is a space in which sustenance can be received. As we come to the end of a single yearly cycle, it is fitting that we dwell, even if only briefly, in the void between one year and the next, letting the full body of the year sink in before we step outside to greet yet another cycle of the earth's journey around the sun. Thus we allow the heart, soul, and spirit to be moved by all we have come to know of the earth's complex and rich personality. Taking this conscious interlude, we can deeply absorb, not through rational understanding, but through skin, bone and heart, the ever-unfolding treasure of this enchanted earth.

SELECTED BIBLIOGRAPHY

Culinary Herbs and Condiments. New York: Dover, 1971

Culpeper's Complete Herbal. London: Bloomsbury Books, 1992

Dawson, Adele. *Herbs: Partners in Life.* Rochester, VT: Healing Arts Press, 1991

Elliot, Doug. *Roots.* Old Greenwich, CT: Chatham Press, 1976

Gladstar, Rosemary. *Herbal Healing For Women.* New York: Fireside Books, Simon & Schuster, 1993

Green, James. *The Male Herbal.* Freedom, CA: The Crossing Press, 1991

Grieves, Maud. *A Modern Herbal.* New York: Dover, 1971

Hopman, Ellen Evert. *Tree Medicine, Tree Magic.* Custer, WA: Phoenix Publishing, 1992.

———. *A Druid's Herbal.* Rochester, VT: Destiny Books, 1995

Levy, Juliette de Baircli. *Common Herbs for Natural Health.* Woodstock, NY: Ashtree Publishing, 1997.

———. *Nature's Children.* (Reprinted by Ashtree Publishing, Woodstock, NY), 1997

Soule, Deb. *The Roots of Healing: A Woman's Book of Herbs.* Secaucus, NJ: Citadel Press, Carol Publishing Group, 1995

———. *Women and Herbs: Exploring our Roots.* Blackberry Books, 1993

Strehlow, Dr. Wighard & Hertzka, Gottfried. *Hildegard's Medicine.* Santa Fe, NM: Bear & Co., 1988

Treben, Maria. *Health Through God's Pharmacy.* Steyr, Austria: Wilhelm Ennsthaler, 1988

Weed, Susun S. *Wise Woman Herbal for the Childbearing Year.* Woodstock, NY: Ashtree Publishing, 1985

———. *Healing Wise* Woodstock, NY: Ashtree Publishing, 1989

———. *Wise Woman Herbal for the Menopausal Years.* Woodstock, NY: Ashtree Publishing, 1992

———. *Breast Cancer? Breast Health! The Wise Woman Way.* Woodstock, NY: Ashtree Publishing, 1997

Wood, Matthew. *The Book of Herbal Wisdom: Using Plants as Medicines.* Berkeley, CA: North Atlantic Books, 1997

MAIL ORDER RESOURCES FOR HERBS

These companies range from small businesses to larger operations. All have fine herbs.

Avena Botanicals, Box 365, West Rockport, ME 04865

Frontier Cooperative Herbs, 3021 78th Street, Norway, IA 52318 (Exceptional blue violet leaf)

Island Herbs c/o Ryan Drum, Waldron Island, WA 98297 (Excellent stinging nettle, red raspberry and kelp flakes)

Jean's Greens, 119 Sulphur Spring Road, Norway, NY 13416 (Excellent variety)

Simpler's Botanicals, P.O. Box 39, Forestville, CA 95436

Woodland Essence, P.O. Box 206, Cold Brook, NY 13324 (family-based business carries fine herbal preparations, including excellent birch body creme)

PLEASE SEND ANY INQUIRIES OR LETTERS TO:

Judith Berger
P.O. Box 1671
Peter Stuyvesant Station
New York, NY 10009

INDEX